Atlas of
Blood and Qi Disorders
in Chinese Medicine

Atlas of

Blood and Qi Disorders

IN CHINESE MEDICINE

氣血

Zhao Jingyi & Li Xuemei

EASTLAND PRESS ▸ SEATTLE

Published by Eastland Press, Inc.
P.O. Box 99749
Seattle, WA 98139, USA
www.eastlandpress.com

Library of Congress Control Number: 2010936723
ISBN: 978-0-939616-72-5
Printed in Korea

2 4 6 8 10 9 7 5 3 1

Brush calligraphy by Xie Keqing
Cover design by Patricia O'Connor
Book design by Gary Niemeier

TABLE OF CONTENTS

FOREWORDS

As qi and blood are basic elements of Chinese medicine, the differentiation of qi and blood disorders is one of the main diagnostic methods. *Atlas of Blood and Qi Disorders in Chinese Medicine* provides photographic images of real cases along with detailed clinical manifestations, diagnostic procedures, treatment principles, and methods. This book will therefore benefit all readers.

I am very honored to introduce the reader to the two authors, Dr Jingyi Zhao and Dr Xuemei Li. Both of them were students of mine over thirty years ago. During their time at the university, they were very dedicated to their studies and their academic achievements were outstanding. Upon graduation, both of them taught and practiced, and following years of hard, day-to-day professional work, they accumulated a great deal of clinical experience and gained a high reputation. This publication is a fine example of their working experience.

Although medical science and diagnostic technologies have developed very rapidly in modern times, traditional Chinese medicine still plays a very important role in the medical field. Its unique diagnostic prinicples, treatment methods, and holistic approach, the use of natural materials to treat the body as an organic whole, and its impressive clinical results have led to its use worldwide. I am delighted to recommend this publication to those in the medical profession as well as students, practitioners and others interested in traditional Chinese medicine.

—Song Tianbin

PROFESSOR AND CHIEF PHYSICIAN, *Beijing University of Chinese Medicine*

VICE PRESIDENT, *International Health Preservation Research Society*

PRESIDENT, *China National Qigong Education and Study Association*

ASSISTANT DIRECTOR OF THE RESEARCH COMMITTEE, *Chinese Health Qigong Association*

CHINESE MEDICAL DIAGNOSIS lies at the core of the practice of acupuncture and Chinese herbal medicine. The traditional ways of diagnosis in the clinic are known to be very difficult to learn and master. I have been teaching acupuncture at universities in the United Kingdom and various Western countries for more than ten years, and am always trying to find the best way to convey this ancient, esoteric knowledge and its associated skills to our students, as Chinese textbooks are not really suitable for the international market. This is not an easy nut to crack, especially when students have little experience in observing patients under supervision.

Professor Zhao and Dr. Li are masters in diagnosis and have been teaching and practicing Chinese medicine for almost thirty years. They have developed their own teaching materials and methods and are very popular among their students.

I know the authors well, as we were college friends at Beijing University of Chinese Medicine, and worked in the same teaching and researching teams for many years before I moved to the University of Lincoln. They have published many titles and their works are highly valued among their peers and students. The names Zhao and Li are familiar to many of my students as they appear in reference lists as the authors of works that are important sources of information.

This new book, together with their other publications, represent a significant contribution to facilitate the understanding of the Chinese method of diagnosis. Photographic images of clinical manifestations are extremely helpful for students, as they avoid the confusion of words or a possible loss of meaning in translation.

It is a pleasure to recommend this book to all readers, practitioners, and practitioners-to-be.

—Meng Fanyi, MB, MM, MATCM

HEAD OF BSC (HONS) ACUPUNCTURE PROGRAMME, *University of Lincoln United Kingdom*

PREFACE

In Chinese medical theory, qi and blood are the most basic elements of the human body and disorders of each can give rise to a number of different conditions, ranging from very mild to very severe. All dysfunctions or abnormalities of the channels, collaterals, and the various tissues or organs of the body are due to changes in the qi and blood. Understanding and treating these particular disorders is extremely important in clinical practice.

Chinese medicine and modern science understand the human body in radically different ways. The concepts of qi and blood, which feature in all Chinese medical books, is often confusing to those who are interested in or studying Chinese medicine. Everyone knows that blood flows through the arteries and veins, but it is difficult to understand why cold blood patterns occur in humans (who are not cold-blooded creatures). The photographs in this book, drawn from actual clinical practice, offer a visual and direct manner of providing answers about patterns of cold blood, hot blood, and blood stasis.

This book addresses the needs of students with a basic knowledge of Chinese medicine, enabling them to master and understand the concepts, clinical symptoms, and physical manifestations of qi and blood disorders. It is suggested that the reader refer to the Appendix ("Additional Information on Qi and Blood") at the end of the book for more details. College lecturers can use this publication as reference source for explaining qi and blood. This book is also useful in defining the eight parameters and organ theory.

For practitioners from different medical backgrounds, the photographs and accompanying text provide a means of understanding some of the differences between Chinese and Western medicine. It is important to realize that a particular disease in Western medicine is not the same thing as a particular pattern in Chinese medicine. Patients can be diagnosed according to Western medicine with a certain disease, but in Chinese medicine the same condition can be diagnosed differently, and vice versa, because Western and traditional Chinese medicine simply use different theoretical systems.

Preface

It is our sincere hope that this book will help readers improve their clinical diagnostic skills.

ACKNOWLEDGMENTS

THE IMAGES IN THIS BOOK have been selected from the photographs that we use as teaching materials. They depict real patients in different hospitals, and were taken over a period of ten years.

We would like to thank all of these patients who kindly allowed us to use the photographs for the purposes of medical education, training doctors, and research. These people firmly believe that if the photographs are put to such use, then others may suffer less than they have. We have been deeply moved to hear such sentiments. Without their understanding, this book could not have been published.

We would like to express our appreciation to our colleagues and university classmates, and to consultants and professors, all working in different specialized fields, from various hospitals. Doctors Huang Li, Xu Yuan, Li Haicong, Song Li, Ji Zhiying and Liu Wali gave us advice based on their own experience, provided us with cases and their typical manifestations, and helped us collect a great deal of clinical information. We would also like to thank doctors Hua Hua and Jiang Yuyong for their help and cooperation.

Once again we are grateful to Charles Gannon, who has helped us with our previous publications. He has devoted much of his time and energy to reading and correcting the English, and has done this in a very thorough manner.

Finally, we greatly appreciate the expert advice and editing provided by John O'Connor, Lilian Bensky, and others at Eastland Press.

CHAPTER 1

Healthy and Unhealthy Appearances

Healthy Complexion

Clinical manifestations

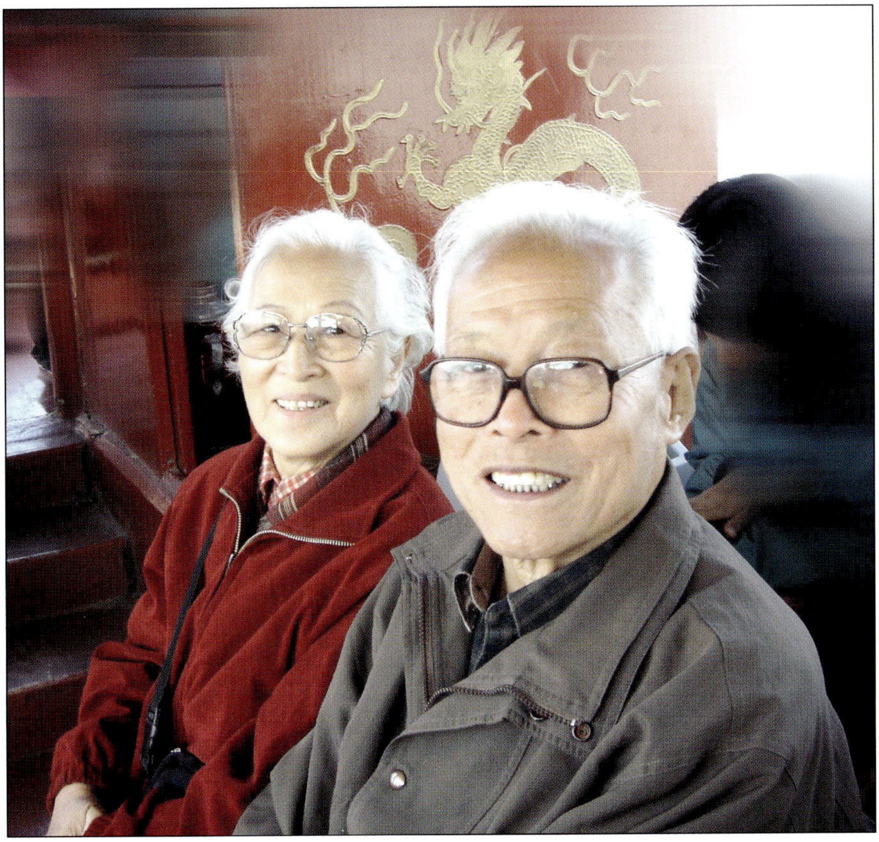

Fig. 1-1: *This image shows people in good health.*

Key points:

A person with normal physiological functions, vigorous in mind and body and free from disease, is regarded as a healthy person. Chinese medicine regards such a person as having a sufficient supply of qi and blood—recognizable from the person's bright eyes, glowing face, keen perception, regular breathing, clear speech, muscular build, and so on.

When disorders of qi and/or blood occur in the body, symptoms emerge which become evidence for diagnosing disease. Many of these symptoms will be reviewed later in this book. In this chapter we will focus on the appearance of the skin, which is very important and readily observable in the clinic.

Examination of the skin, as well as the complexion of the face, includes the color and the general appearance of the skin. The color of the skin refers to both skin tone, which, depending on race and region, may be white, brown or black, and also a lighter or darker change in the basic skin color. The general appearance of the skin refers to its other characteristics, such as luster and moisture, which reflect its nourishment and serve as evidence in understanding the condition of qi and blood in the body.

The color of the complexion or skin is a mixture of the basic color of the skin itself together with a light rosy color, a manifestation of blood circulation in the body as it nourishes the skin and thus appears as a rosy hue through the skin.

The general appearance of the complexion or skin includes its luster or shine, elasticity (skin turgor) and moisture, which are linked to age, gender, and the effects of the environment, as well as the nourishment of the skin, which is supplied by qi and blood in the body. These factors are not linked to skin color. By this we mean that, no matter the race or color, the general appearance of the skin and face can be judged by the same standard if the state of health is similar.

In Chinese medicine a normal complexion for Chinese people would be described as light brown mixed with pink, with normal moisture and luster. Similarly, those with white, brown, or black skin mixed with pink or rosiness (reflecting blood in the skin), together with normal moisture and luster, would be considered normal. (See Ch. 3 on blood deficiency for further detail.)

Diagnosis

A healthy complexion reflects sufficient qi and blood, and efficient antipathogenic factors.

Abnormal Appearance

Clinical manifestations

The following images are of different types of patients seen in the clinic.

Key points: See Figs. 1-2 through 1-5 (pp. 3-4).

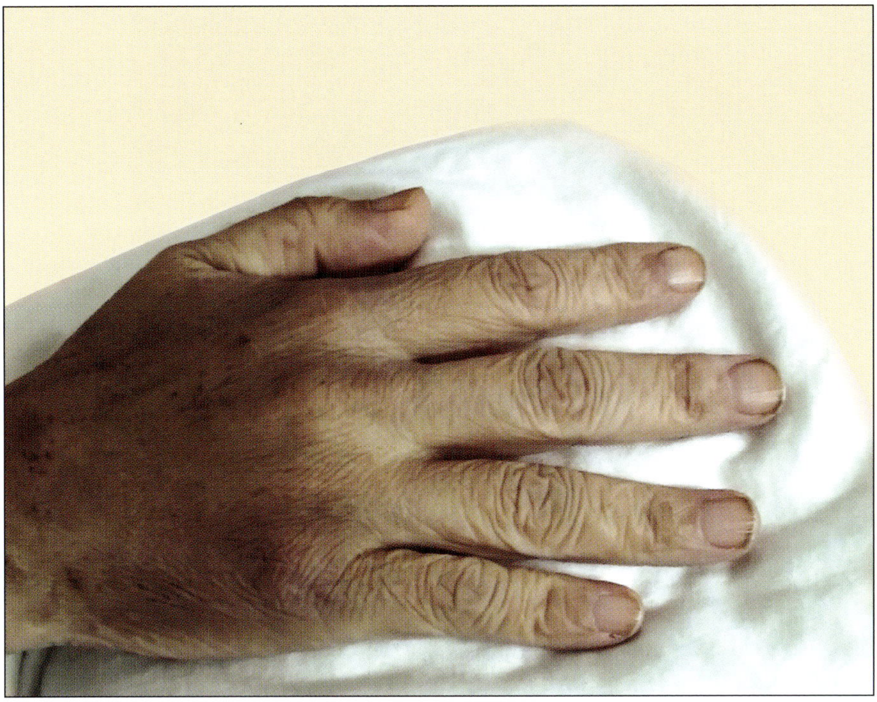

Fig. 1-2: *Pale skin with reduced elasticity*

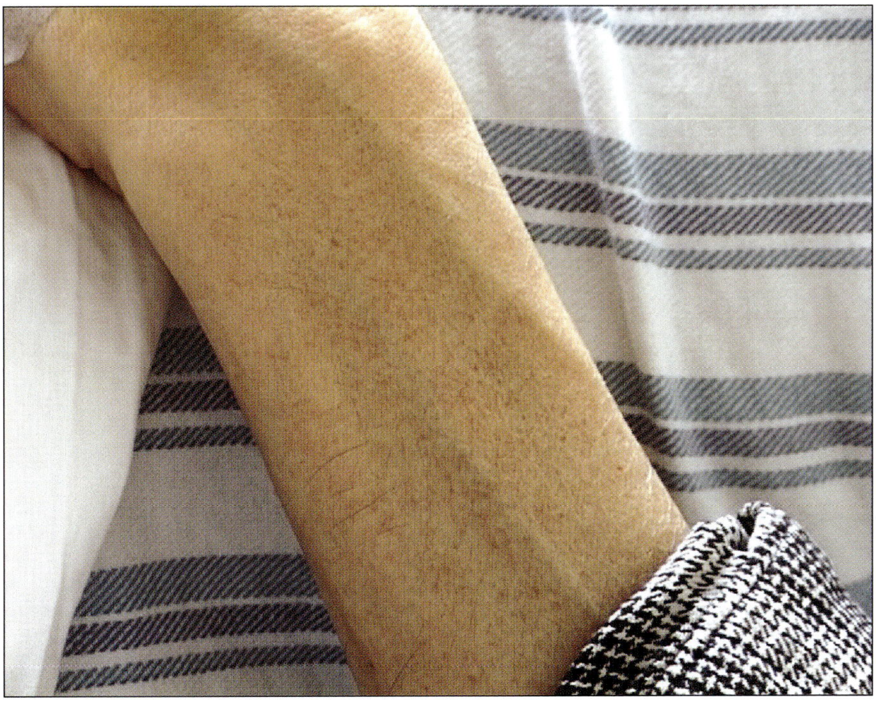

Fig. 1-3: *Dry and lusterless skin*

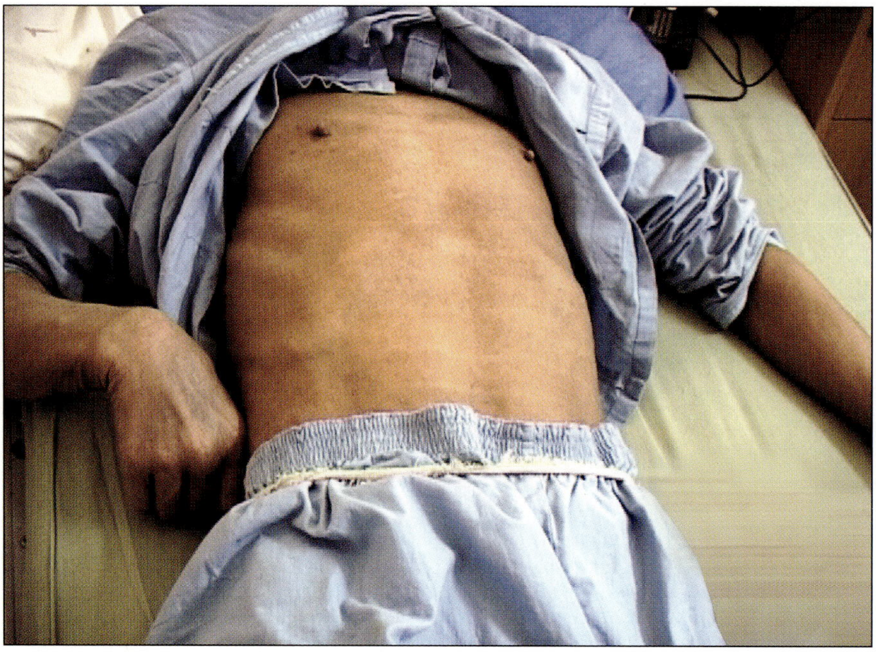

Fig. 1-4: *Dusky, lusterless skin and generalized hyperpigmentation*
The skin looks as though the body has been unwashed for a long time.

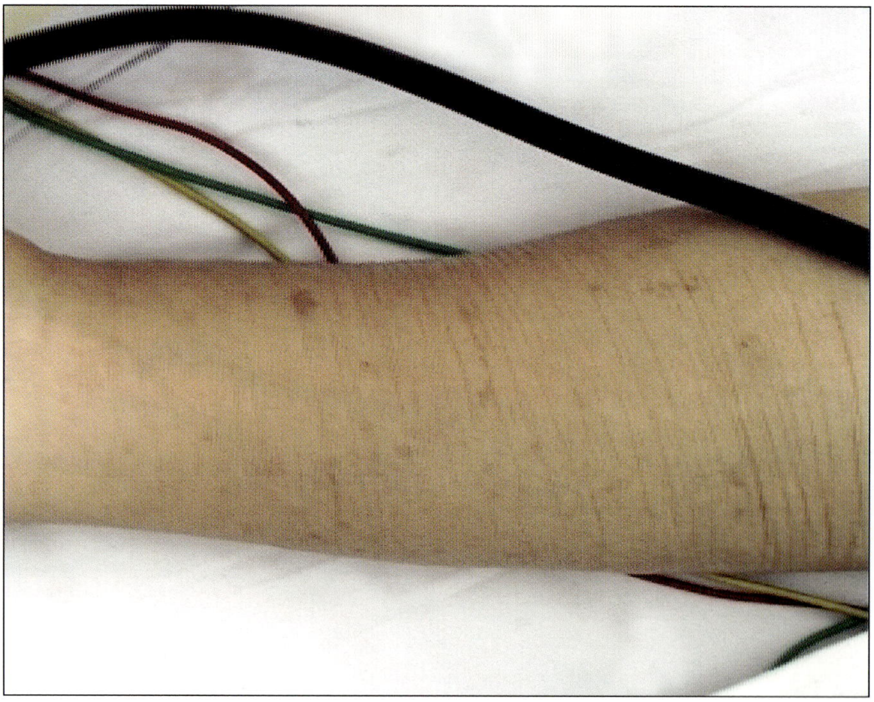

Fig. 1-5: *Dusky and lusterless skin and wrinkles on the forearm*
These signs result from very poor elasticity (poor skin turgor).

Pathological process

As noted above, the color and general appearance of the skin need to be diagnosed separately in the clinic. Some abnormal appearances of the skin will be detailed in this section.

In general, vitality is present in all living things: human beings, animals, and plants. It is easy to differentiate between living things with vitality and those without life force or vitality. For example, luxuriant vegetation and withered plants are very different because the former has vitality and the latter does not.

Skin likewise shows a clear indication of life force. The appearance of the skin is closely associated with a person's state of health or with the severity of a disease, that is, with the sufficiency or insufficiency of the qi and blood. The images shown here are from patients suffering from different diseases. All have poor skin appearance, especially the lack of luster, indicating an insufficiency of qi and blood which causes malnourishment not only of the skin, but of the entire body. Fig. 1-5 reveals a severely diseased patient in the late stage of illness. The dusky, lusterless, and wrinkled skin indicates a deficiency of qi and blood (the antipathogenic factors), which are extremely exhausted by both the long-term disease and the pathogenic factors.

Diagnosis

Injury to the qi and blood

The difference in the appearance of the skin is closely related to the condition of the qi and blood in the body, and so we are able to make a diagnosis.

Comparison

Clinical manifestations

These images compare the appearance of the skin in healthy people vs. unhealthy patients.

Key Points: See Figs. 1-6 and 1-7 (p. 6).

Diagnosis

This chapter provides a general principle for identifying the state of the patient's health (also the qi and blood) based on the appearance of the skin. It is applicable to all patients that one sees in the clinic.

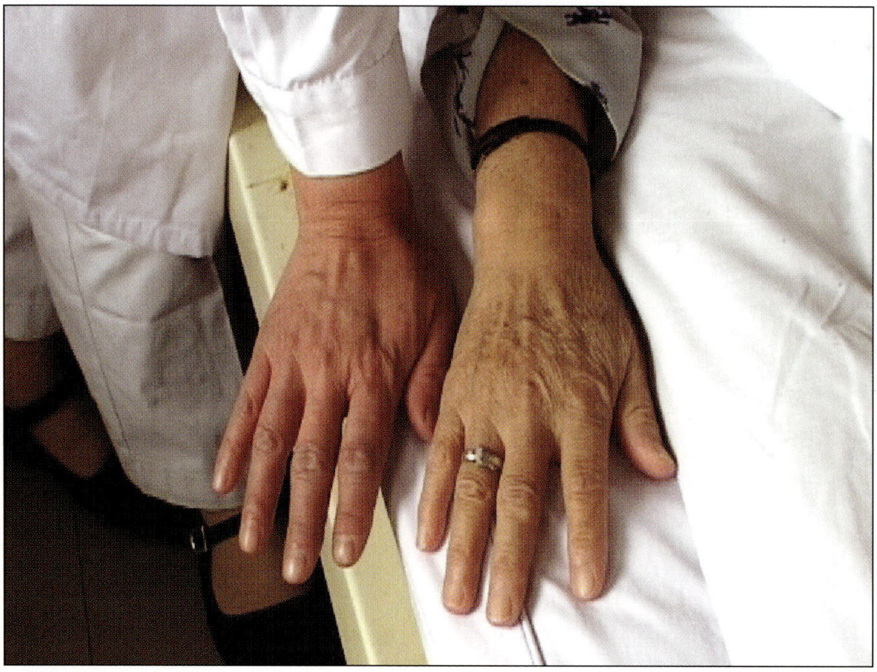

Fig. 1-6: *The normal skin of a physician compared with that of a patient*

The color and general appearance of the skin are quite different.

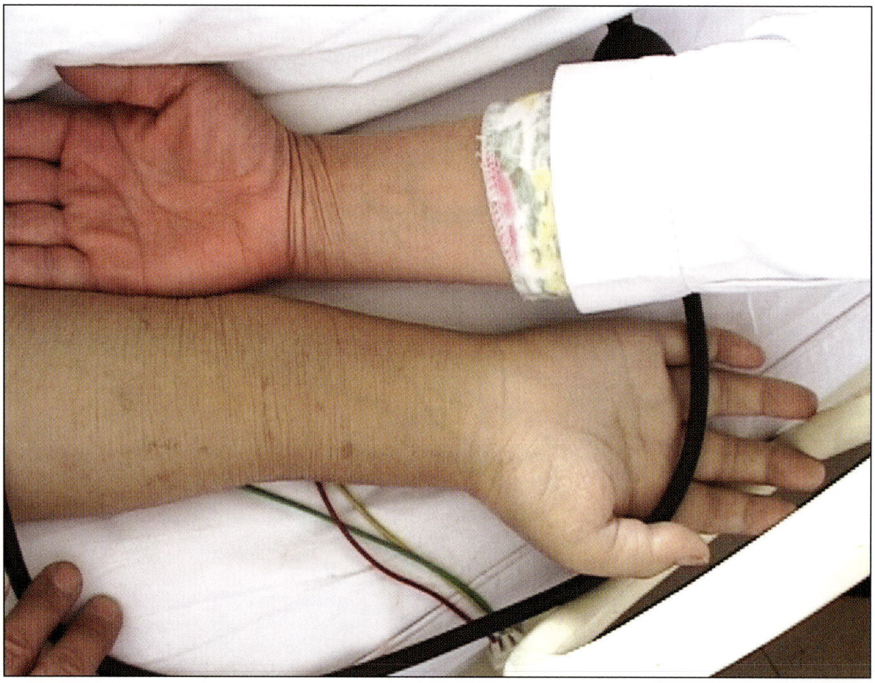

Fig. 1-7: *The same patient seen in Fig. 1-5 compared with a doctor's arm*

The color and general appearance of the skin are quite different.

CHAPTER 2

Patterns of Qi Deficiency

(Spleen Qi Deficiency and Spleen Yang Deficiency)

Sallow or Pale Skin

Clinical manifestations

Sallow or pale skin, body emaciation, and weakness

Key points: See Figs. 2-1 through 2-3 (below and p. 8).

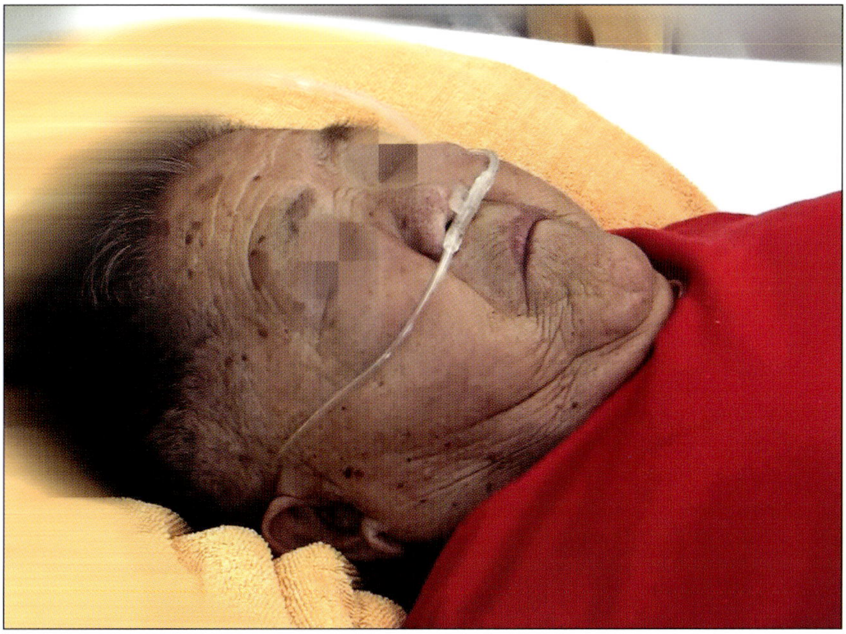

Fig. 2-1: *Heart failure*

The patient's complexion is sallow, dry, lusterless, wrinkled, and has poor elasticity.

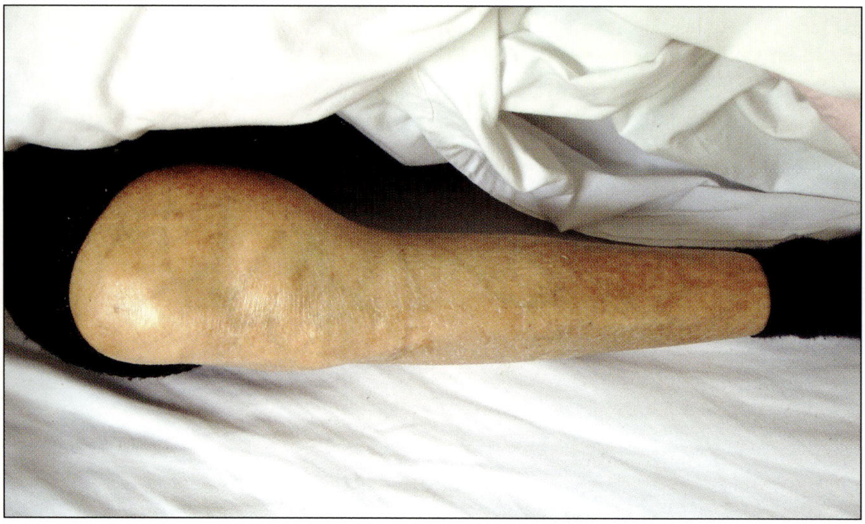

Fig. 2-2: *Cerebrovascular disease*
The legs are emaciated and the skin is sallow.

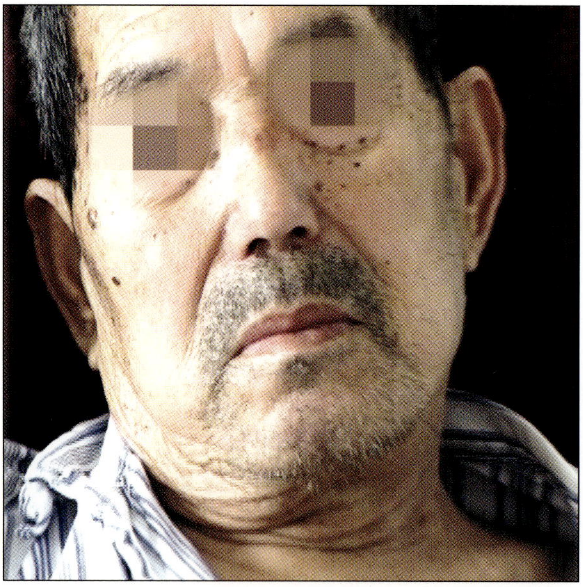

Fig. 2-3: *Obstructive pulmonary emphysema*
The complexion is pale.

Pathological process

Sallowness or paleness indicates malnourishment of the skin.

According to Chinese medicine, the skin is nourished and colored by vital essence and blood, both of which emanate from food. The middle burner (Spleen and Stomach) is the source of postnatal nutrition and fills an important function in transforming the food into food essence and blood.

Dysfunction of the Spleen leads to insufficient production of food essence, which can directly cause malnourishment of the skin, resulting in sallowness. Meanwhile the reduced blood production leads to blood deficiency, which causes the skin to lose its rosy bloom, moisture, and nourishment, becoming pale and dry and with reduced elasticity.

Another manifestation of malnourishment is the loss of normal volume in the muscles, which explains why patients become emaciated. (See Figs. 2-4 through 2-7 for more details.)

Diagnosis

Spleen deficiency

Sallow or pale skin indicates that the site of the disease is the Spleen. Dry, sagging, withered skin (Fig. 2-1) that lacks normal luster and has poor elasticity indicates malnourishment of the skin. Notably emaciated lower limbs (Fig. 2-2) indicate that the Spleen deficiency is quite severe and the muscles have obviously lost their nourishment.

Differential diagnosis

Sallow or pale skin is a common condition when there is Spleen deficiency.

Spleen qi deficiency or Spleen yang deficiency can both result in the skin undergoing similar changes. Spleen qi deficiency is often the cause of the skin becoming sallow while Spleen yang deficiency is more likely to produce a pale appearance. This is because Spleen yang deficiency weakens the water metabolism and the ensuing dampness remains in the body, which affects the skin and presents as a pale color.

A similar change in skin color can also be observed in patterns of dual qi and blood deficiency because Spleen qi deficiency very commonly leads to blood deficiency. (For more detail, see Ch. 3 on blood deficiency.

Emaciated Muscles

Clinical manifestations

Emaciation, that is, loss of weight or mass and volume of the muscles of the entire body or a part of the body or a limb.

Key points: See Figs. 2-4 through 2-7 (pp. 10-11).

Pathological process

Emaciation indicates that the muscles lack sufficient nutrition. The body absorbs nourishment from food in order to supply the body yin and yang. Strength pertains to the yang aspect of the body, which is supported by the yang of nature and food, while the body itself (its muscles, bones, organs, skin, and so forth) pertains to the

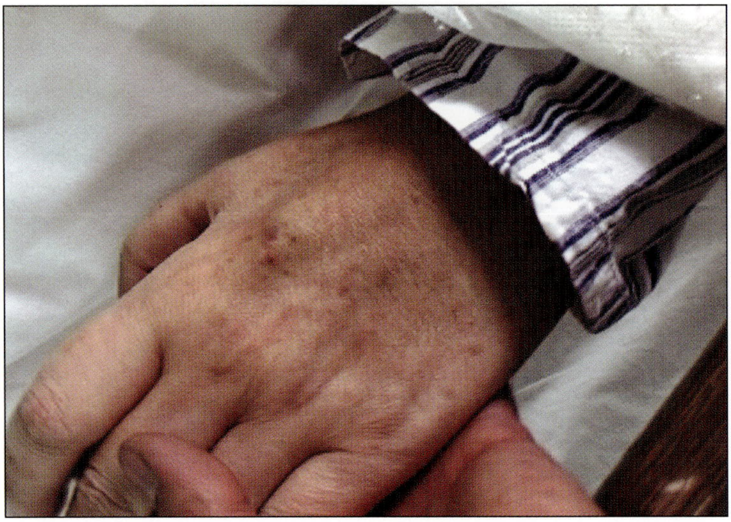

Fig. 2-4: *Amyotrophic lateral sclerosis (ALS)*

The patient has muscular atrophy of the hand (atrophy of the dorsal interossei and thenar muscles). The skin is pale.

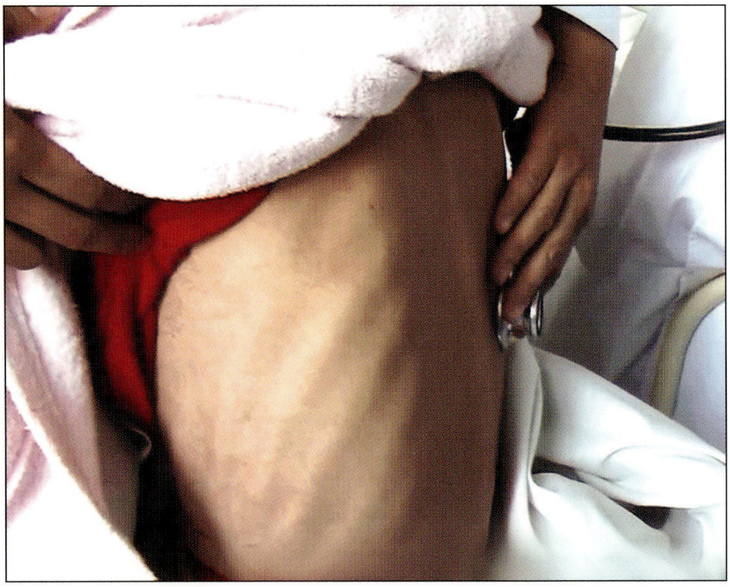

Fig. 2-5: *Renal failure with uremia*

This is the same patient shown in Figs. 3-4 and 3-5 in the following chapter on blood deficiency. The patient is severely emaciated. The shape of the bones can be distinguished and the ribs and spine can be clearly seen.

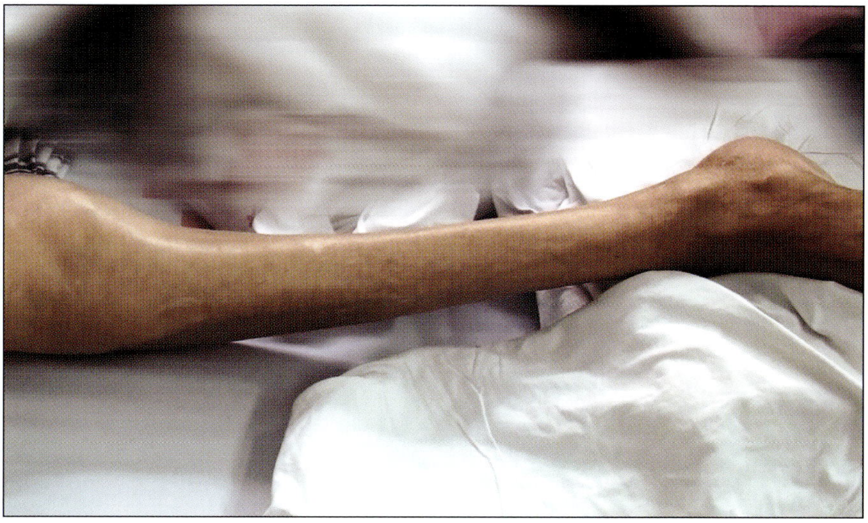

Fig. 2-6: *Cerebrovascular disease*

The skin is sallow and the legs are extremely thin and not significantly wider than their supporting bones.

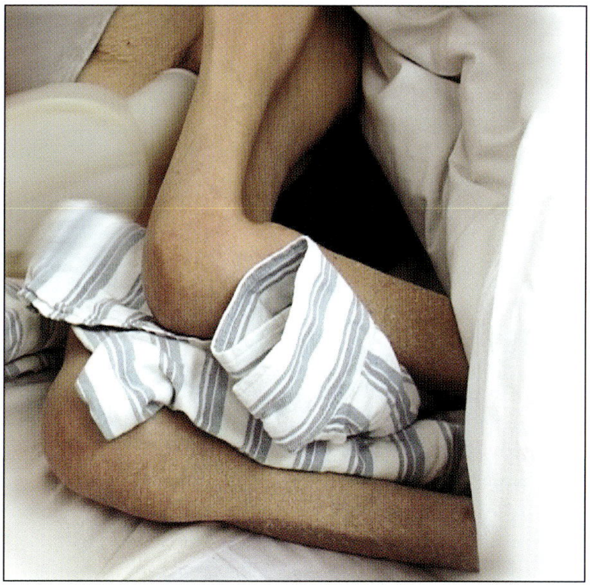

Fig. 2-7: *Advanced cancer*

The major muscles of the lower limbs are very emaciated; the skin is pale and lusterless.

yin aspect of the body, which is supplied by food essence. Muscles pertain to the yin aspect of the body and benefit from food essence.

A patient with Spleen deficiency, which leads to a dysfunction in one's transporting and transforming capacity, becomes thin because food essence cannot be produced properly. The shortage of food essence causes malnourishment of the muscles, which thereupon become emaciated.

Insufficiency in the production of food essence also leads to a reduction in the generation of blood. The skin loses its normal nourishment from the blood and thus becomes pale or sallow and lusterless.

Diagnosis

Spleen deficiency, which leads to malnourishment of the body

Pale or sallow skin indicates malnourishment of the skin caused by a deficiency of qi and blood. Emaciation of the body and limbs indicates malnourishment of the muscles.

Differential diagnosis

Loss of volume of the muscles, that is, emaciation, is an important diagnostic indication of Spleen deficiency. Located at the extremities of the body, the hands and feet receive less nourishment of qi, blood, and food essence than other parts of the body, and are thus most at risk for manifestations of malnutrition.

The muscles of the hands are often atrophied at an early stage of illness. Comparatively bigger muscles, such as those of the thighs and buttocks, usually become atrophied only at a later stage, reflecting the severity of the Spleen deficiency.

Exhaustion or Weakness

Clinical manifestations

Emaciated limbs and weakened movements. Patients feel fatigued and become tired easily, and may not even be able to sit or stand up. The symptoms worsen with physical activity. Slurred speech and dysphagia may be manifested.

Key points: See Figs. 2-8 and 2-9 (p. 13).

Pathological process

The weakness of the muscles is a manifestation of the deficiency of Spleen qi.

According to Chinese medicine, the Spleen governs the muscles and limbs, which means that both the substance and strength of the muscles and limbs are associated with the Spleen. As noted earlier, the muscles themselves benefit from food essence but their ability to extend and contract is supported by the qi, which is also derived from the Spleen, and enables them to carry out their normal activities.

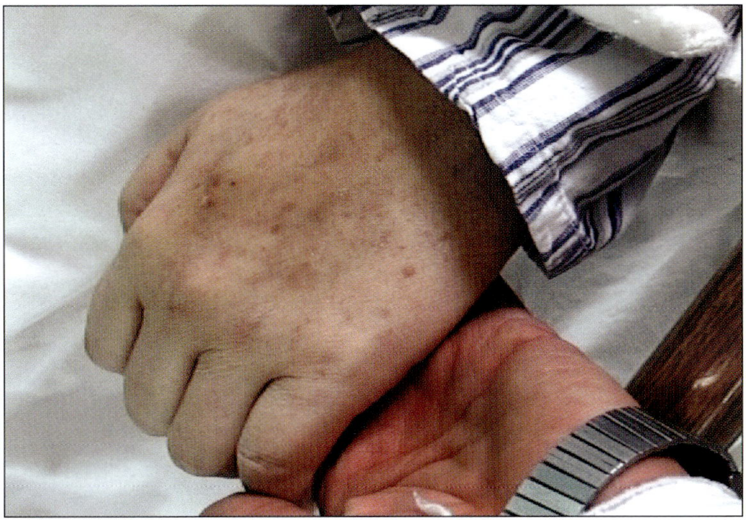

Fig. 2-8: *Amyotrophic lateral sclerosis (ALS)*

This is the same patient shown in Fig. 2-4. The patient is unable to move his hands and fingers. The skin of the patient's hand is pale compared to that of the doctor's hand.

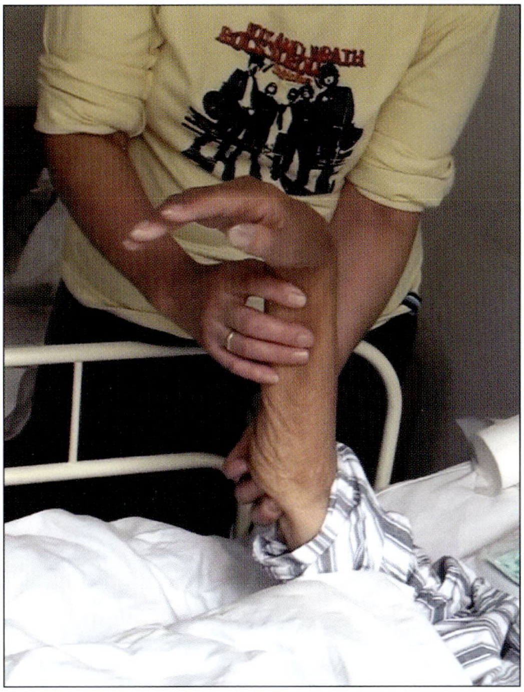

Fig. 2-9: *Paralysis due to stroke*

The patient is emaciated. The right arm droops and there is complete loss of muscle function, rendering it immovable. The skin is sallow.

Qi deficiency results in reduced physical energy such that the movement of the limbs is weak or nonexistent. Because the muscles are so weak, the limbs can no longer be held in an active position and the hands droop. Spleen deficiency leads to emaciation and a loss of normal muscle volume.

The diminished production of food essence leads to malnourishment of the skin, which becomes pale and lacks a normal luster.

Diagnosis

Spleen qi deficiency causes reduced strength and leads to weakness of the limbs.

Emaciated and softened hands indicate Spleen qi deficiency, which cannot maintain the normal shape of the muscles. Weakness of limb movement reflects insufficient Spleen qi strength in the limbs, that is, the energy (qi) is very weak.

Differential diagnosis

Adequate muscle volume is closely related to the food essence. If there is a dysfunction in the Spleen's ability to transport and transform food, the muscles will become emaciated, as noted above and shown in Figs. 2-4 through 2-7.

On the other hand, physical movement or its absence (exhaustion or weakness) is mainly related to the strength that is supplied by the Spleen qi. Clinically, generalized fatigue or easily becoming tired is a common manifestation of Spleen qi deficiency. Unfortunately, tiredness and fatigue are subjective symptoms and do not appear in photographs. The images seen here are of severe cases of Spleen qi deficiency, which are regarded as patterns of atrophy disorder (*wěi zhèng* 痿证) in Chinese medicine.

Edema

Clinical manifestations

Pitting edema in the skin, most commonly seen on the lower limbs. Heavy, distending sensation and fatigue are common complaints. The skin may appear stretched and even shiny in its puffiness.

Key points: See Figs. 2-10 through 2-12 (pp. 15-16).

Pathological process

Edema is a result of impaired water metabolism.

The Spleen is one of the organs responsible for water metabolism and its malfunction is one of the most common reasons for edema. When the Spleen qi is deficient, its function of transporting and transforming water, as well as dampness, is weakened; the metabolism of water is therefore weak. The ensuing water can accumulate in the skin, leading to edema. The natural tendency of water is to sink and therefore the edema often appears in the lower part of the body.

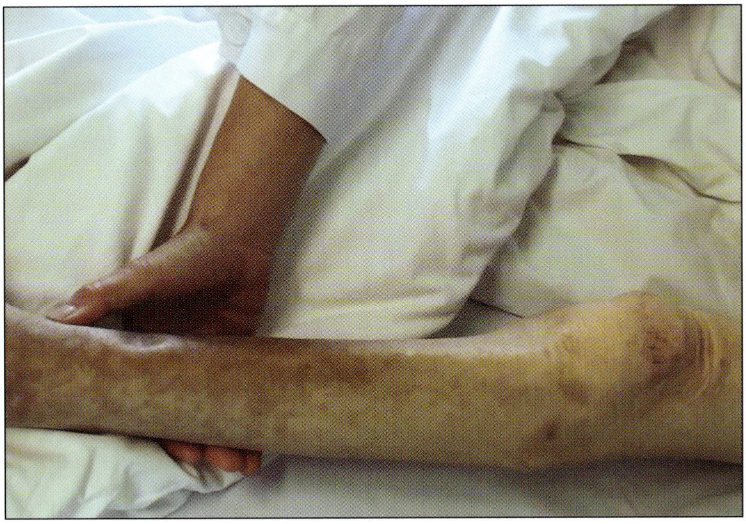

Fig. 2-10: *Heart failure*

This is the same patient shown in Fig. 2-1, who has edema in the lower limbs. The patient has a suffocating sensation in the chest and shortness of breath. These symptoms worsen with physical activity.

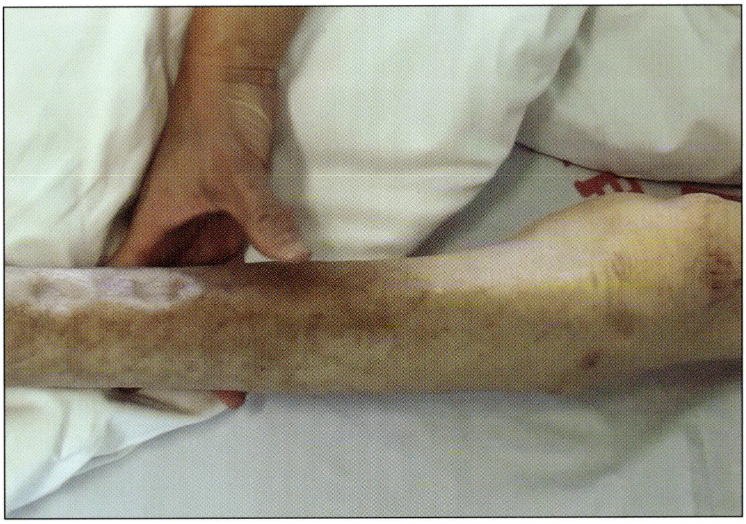

Fig. 2-11: *Heart failure*

This again is the patient with edema of the leg. Finger pressure on the leg leaves pits or depressions, which return to normal after a few seconds.

Symptoms such as shortness of breath and a suffocating sensation in the chest prove that there is also a pattern of Lung qi deficiency; the Lung qi's function of dispersing and descending cannot be performed properly.

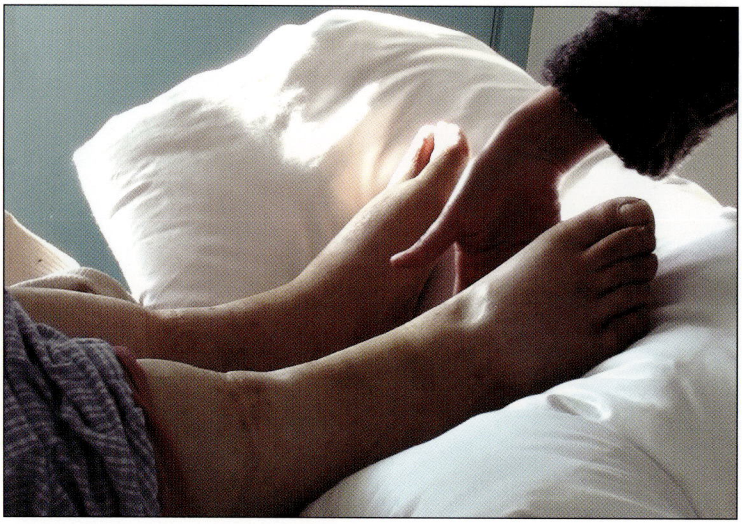

Fig. 2-12: *Chronic liver disease*
The patient has edema of the feet, with pitting.

Diagnosis

Spleen deficiency leads to a retention of pathogenic water as well as Lung qi deficiency.

Edema indicates Spleen deficiency and a retention of water in the skin. That the symptoms become more severe following physical activity also indicates qi deficiency. The suffocating sensation in the chest, as well as shortness of breath, indicate Lung qi deficiency.

Differential diagnosis

According to the theory of five phases, the Spleen pertains to the earth phase and the Lung to metal, thus the Spleen and Lung have a generating (mother-son) relationship. Additionally, the Lung governs the qi and the Spleen is the source of the qi. The Lung and Spleen have a close physiological relationship: if one becomes diseased it will often affect the other. In the clinic, qi deficiency of both the Spleen and Lung is very common. Because the treatment of both is the same, it is unnecessary to determine which is the original cause of disease.

Ascites

Clinical manifestations

Fullness and distention of the abdomen, bodily emaciation, poor appetite and fatigue, being bedridden

Key points: See Figs. 2-13 and 2-14 (p. 17).

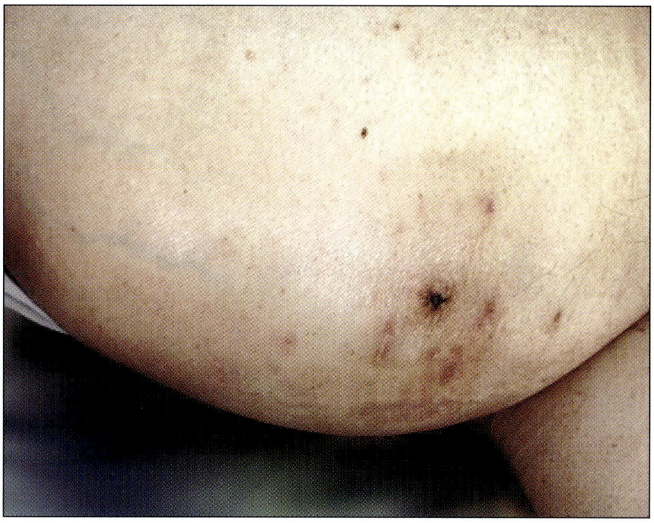

Fig. 2-13: *Advanced stage of cancer with ascites*

The patient has fullness and distention, swollen abdomen, and visibly distended veins beneath the skin.

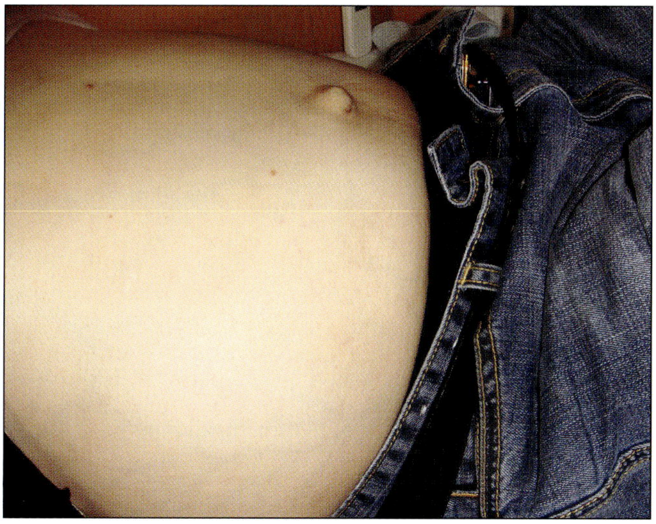

Fig.2-14: *Alcoholic cirrhosis and ascites*

The abdomen is markedly distended with pronounced umbilical distention.

Pathological process

Ascites is the manifestation of a build-up of pathogenic water in the abdominal (peritoneal) cavity.

The functions of Spleen qi and yang are to transport and transform water into body fluids. Pathogenic water is associated with yin and can block the circulation of qi in the middle burner, readily injuring the yang qi of the Spleen and Stomach. The retention of pathogenic water, originally caused by the Spleen's malfunction, can aggravate this condition. Symptoms such as fullness and discomfort in the abdomen, distended abdominal cavity, and even pronounced umbilical distention can develop.

The normal function of Spleen qi is diminished and the food cannot properly be transformed into essence, leading to a lack of energy and poor appetite followed by fatigue and emaciation.

The antipathogenic factors have been badly damaged by a long period of illness, marking a severe stage of the disease.

The enlarged veins (Fig. 2-13) indicate that there is blood stasis. See Ch. 6 on blood stasis for more details.

Diagnosis

Spleen deficiency in which there is both Spleen qi and yang deficiency, together with blood stasis and qi stagnation and retention of pathogenic water

The abdominal discomfort and fullness indicate qi stagnation and retention of pathogenic water in the abdominal cavity. Emaciation and fatigue indicate Spleen deficiency. The enlarged veins visible through the skin reflect the presence of blood stasis.

Differential diagnosis

Compared with the previous group of images (Figs. 2-10 through 2-12), it is clear that they have similar pathological processes: Spleen deficiency and impaired water metabolism. The difference is that in the edema group (Figs. 2-10 through 2-12), Spleen deficiency produces water, which is a pattern of deficiency. On the other hand, in the ascites group (Figs. 2-13, 2-14), the pathogenic water interferes with the Spleen qi and yang, which are already damaged, and thus there is a pattern of deficiency and excess.

There are similar cases in Ch. 6 (blood stasis) because both involve severe blood stasis and retention of pathogenic water.

Loose Stools

Clinical manifestations

Recurrent diarrhea caused by the intake of improper food or induced by tiredness or overwork. The abdomen feels uncomfortable and patients suffer from poor appetite and fatigue.

Key points: See Figs. 2-15 and 2-16 (p. 19).

Pathological process

Soft or loose stools indicate a malfunction in the transportation and transformation of food by the Spleen. The function of the Spleen is to transform and transport food.

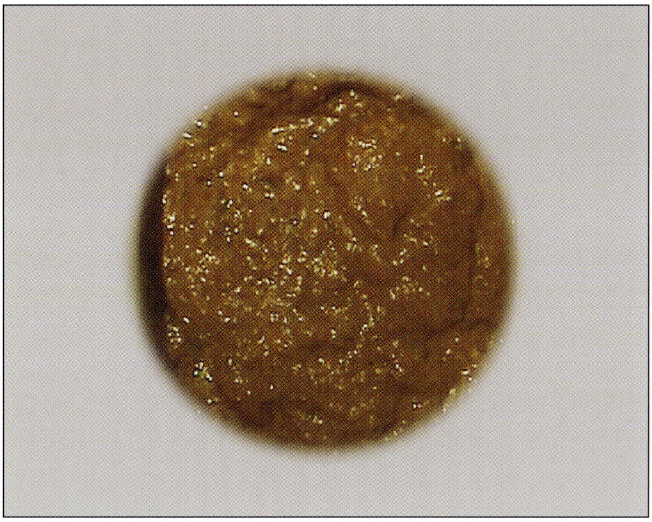

Fig. 2-15: *Chronic diarrhea*

This is soft, unformed, sticky feces with bright reflective spots, which indicate that they contain too much liquid. No blood or pus is present.

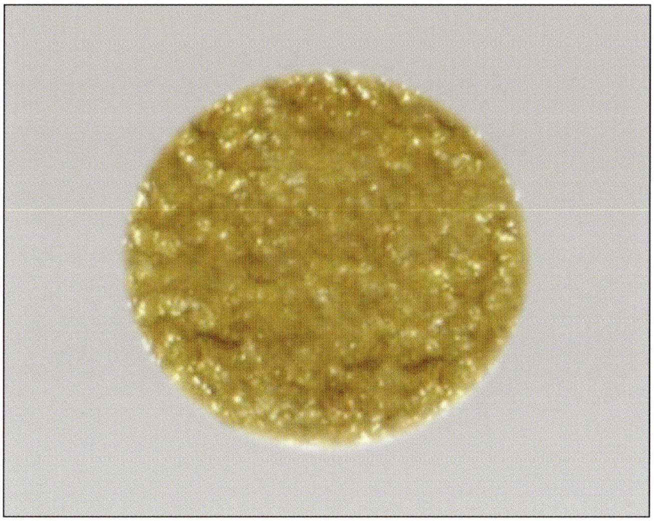

Fig. 2-16: *Another case of chronic diarrhea*

These are unformed stools, looser than in Fig. 2-15, but not watery. The color is normal.

The transformation process involves the breakdown of food into nutritive essence (or food essence), which pertains to clear yang, and which is raised up to the Lung and spread thoughout the entire body to nourish the organs. The remaining turbid part of the food is waste, which pertains to turbid yin, and is transported into the Large Intestine as feces.

Because of Spleen deficiency, the food essence cannot be properly extracted from the food and becomes mixed with the waste. The mixture of food essence and waste enters the Large Intestine and causes sticky and unformed stools.

If the water metabolism has also been damaged, that is, the body fluids are not properly transported by the Spleen, they descend to the Large Intestine where they cause looser stools.

Diagnosis

Spleen deficiency causes a failure in the separation of clear yang and turbid waste from the food.

Unformed and sticky stools (Fig. 2-15) indicate Spleen qi deficiency, which leads to the mixing of clear yang and turbid yin. Unformed and looser stools (Fig. 2-16) indicate Spleen yang deficiency, which causes the extra water to descend to the Large Intestine. Diarrhea caused by the intake of improper food or induced by tiredness or overwork, as well as poor appetite and fatigue, are all indicative of Spleen deficiency.

Differential diagnosis

The cause of diarrhea, which may be pathogenic factors or a malfunction of the organs, can be ascertained by examining the features of the stool.

Spleen deficiency, including Spleen qi deficiency and Spleen yang deficiency, are its common causes and can be differentiated by observing the features of the stools, as noted above.

Watery stools indicate Kidney yang deficiency because they contain too much water.

Stools containing blood and mucus imply an invasion by damp-heat of the Large Intestine, which is commonly caused by the environment or contaminated food. If the stools contain particles of undigested food, there is either food retention or, in certain circumstances, Kidney yang deficiency.

Prolapsed Organs

Clinical manifestations

Drooping eyelids, prolapse of the rectum or uterus, or prolapse of internal organs in the abdomen

Key points: See Figs. 2-17 and 2-18 (p. 21).

Pathological process

Drooping eyelids or prolapse of the organs is the clinical manifestation of a failure of clear yang qi to rise.

Qi pertains to yang and has a tendency to rise, just like hot air in nature. In a healthy body, there is sufficient qi (or sufficient clear yang qi) to rise upward and hold

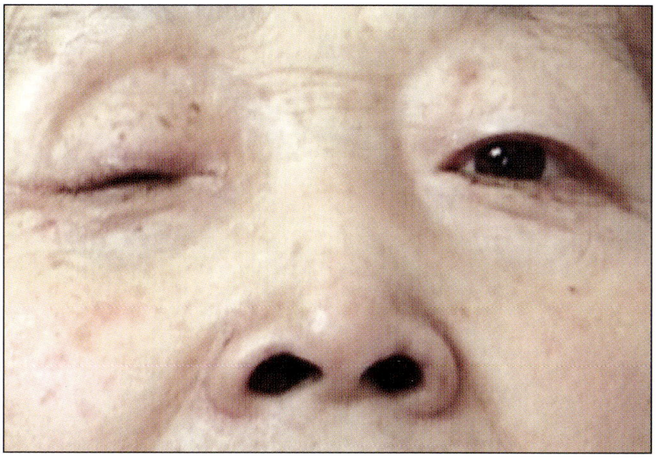

Fig. 2-17: *Drooping eyelid*
The right eyelid is drooping and the patient has difficulty opening it.

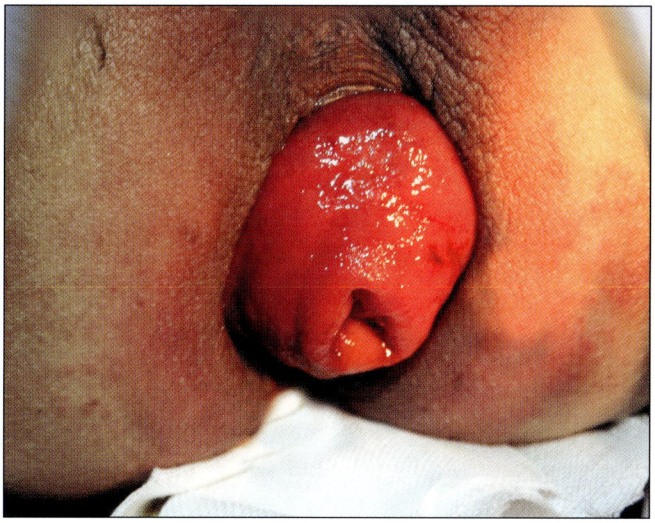

Fig. 2-18: *Rectal prolapse*
This is the protrusion of the rectum through the anus.
The dark red membranous surface of the rectum is visible.

the organs in their proper positions. Qi deficiency, especially Spleen qi deficiency, weakens both the ability of qi to rise as well as its holding action; because the energy that keeps the organs in their normal positions has failed, it has led in this case to the prolapse of the rectum.

In Chinese medicine, the eyelid is associated with the Spleen because of the muscles that are governed by it. Because of Spleen qi deficiency, the function of supporting the eyelid is impaired such that the patient has difficulty opening the eyelid.

Diagnosis

Spleen deficiency resulting in failure of the clear yang qi to rise

A drooping eyelid indicates a weakness of the muscles, which is caused by Spleen qi deficiency. Prolapse of the rectum is evidence of a weakness of the clear yang qi in rising, which is also caused by Spleen qi deficiency.

Differential diagnosis

Failure of the clear yang qi to rise (*qīng yáng bù shēng* 清阳不升) or sunken Spleen qi (*pí qì xià xiàn* 脾气下陷), associated with Spleen qi deficiency, can cause various organs (the Stomach, Liver, or Kidney) to lose their normal positions within the body; the eyelids can droop, and the rectum and uterus can become prolapsed. Although the symptoms are different, the pathological process is the same: all are caused by poor energy being unable to raise the clear yang due to Spleen deficiency.

Hemorrhage

Clinical manifestations

Recurrent hemorrhage with a pale or sallow, weak, and lusterless appearance. Patients often complain of shortness of breath, dizziness, fatigue, and tiredness.

Key points: See Fig. 2-19 below.

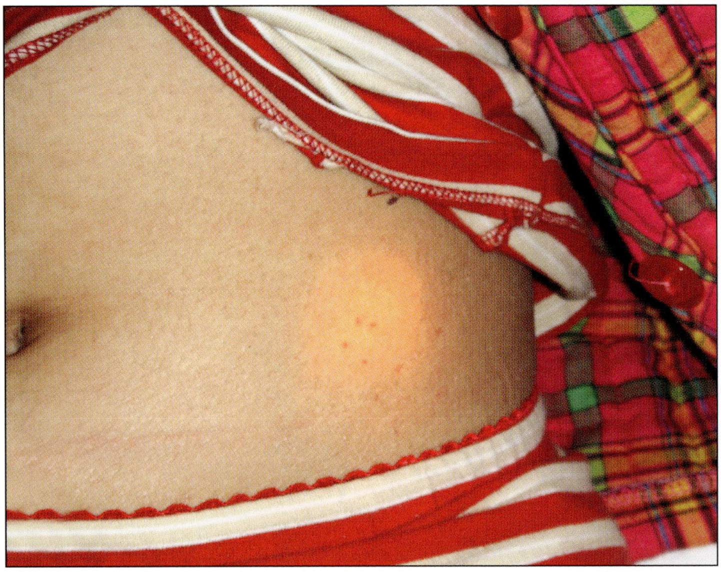

Fig. 2-19: *Idiopathic thrombocytopenic purpura (ITP)*

A small group of pinpoint light red spots (petechiae) have appeared on the illuminated area of abdominal skin. The color of the petechiae does not disappear after pressure is applied to the area and the skin is pale and lusterless. (See Ch. 7 on bleeding for more details.)

Gum Disease

Clinical manifestations

Advanced stages of periodontitis. The gums are significantly destroyed and bleed easily. The gums may have pulled away from the teeth and receded. The teeth may begin to loosen.

Key points: See Figs. 2-20 and 2-21 (p. 24).

Pathological process

Seriously damaged gums and the surrounding tissue that support the teeth indicate a significant loss of support from the essence of the middle burner.

In Chinese medicine the gums are closely associated, through the yang brightness channel, with the Stomach and Spleen. These are the main organs in the middle burner and are the source of qi and blood production. Deficiency of qi in the Stomach and Spleen leads to a dysfunction in transportation and transformation and can also cause a deficiency of blood, resulting in a pattern of both blood and qi deficiency. The images here show evidence of this.

Fig. 2-21 shows that most of the gums have been affected and that changes have occurred in both the color and the texture of the gums due to the deficiency of blood and qi. In Fig. 2-20, only a few teeth have been affected but the destruction of the gums is more obvious—evidence that the Spleen qi deficiency is more severe.

Diagnosis

Thin or receded gums indicate that the patient has a deficiency of qi in the Spleen and Stomach, leading to a dysfunction of transportation and transformation, and thus the gums lose their normal nourishment from the essence of food.

Pale color indicates that there is also blood deficiency.

Differential diagnosis

Periodontal disease is a chronic process with different stages. The early stage is usually characterized by inflammation, experienced as tenderness, redness, and puffiness around the teeth. At this stage, Stomach fire is more likely considered because it can ascend along the yang brightness channel. The advanced stage of periodontitis is connected with more qi deficiency than Stomach fire, and symptoms of pale, thin, and receded gums are more evident than red and swollen gums.

Pale Tongue with Teeth Marks

A pale, swollen, and flabby tongue with teeth marks around the border is a typical manifestation on the tongue of qi deficiency, especially with a pattern of Spleen qi or yang deficiency. For more information, please refer to the section on tongue diagnosis.

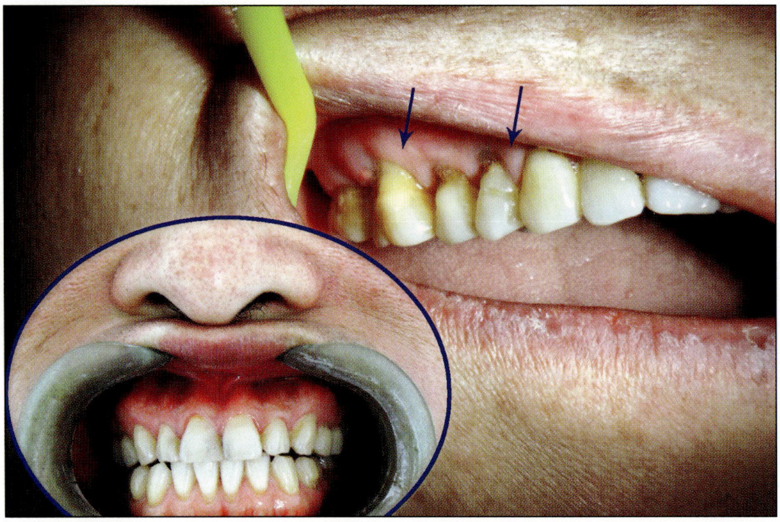

Fig. 2-20: *Periodontal disease*

Compared with healthy gums (displayed at the bottom left corner), the patient's gums have receded and thus some of the teeth look longer because the gums have been destroyed.

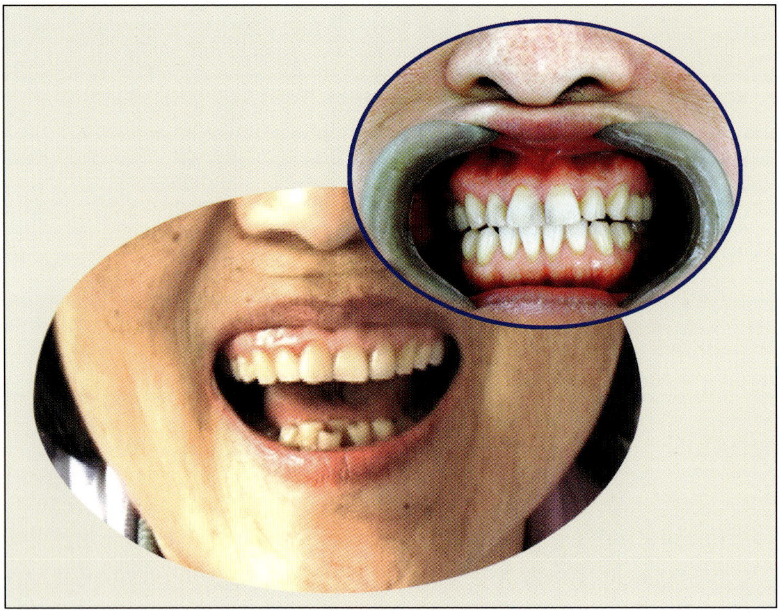

Fig. 2-21: *Iron deficiency anemia*

The gums have lost their normal coral pink color, as shown on the upper right of the photo, and have become pale and thin.

Summary

Table 2-1: *Key diagnostic points for patterns of qi and Spleen deficiency*

Underlying Cause	Symptoms (Images)	Examples of Diseases and Symptoms
Malnourishment of the skin	Sallow complexion and withered skin (Figs. 2-1 to 2-3)	Anemia (e.g., aplastic anemia); malnutrition (e.g., rickets, chronic disease); recovery from disease or surgery
Dysfunction of the Spleen's transportation and transformation	Poor appetite and abdominal discomfort	Digestive diseases (e.g., chronic gastritis); disorders associated with delayed gastric emptying; recovery from disease
	Abdominal pain that can be relieved by pressure; diarrhea or loose stools (Figs. 2-15 and 2-16)	Digestive disorders (e.g., gastro-intestinal spasm, chronic diarrhea, colitis, irritable bowel syndrome)
Malnourishment of the muscles	Emaciation, fatigue or tiredness, lassitude (Figs. 2-4 to 2-9)	Malnutrition (e.g., malabsorption syndromes); motor neuron diseases (e.g., amyotrophic lateral sclerosis [ALS]); neuromuscular disorder (e.g., multiple sclerosis [MS]); malignant conditions (e.g., cancer, cachexia)
	Gum disease (Figs. 2-20 to 2-21)	Periodontal disease (e.g., periodontitis)
Retention of pathogenic water	Edema (Figs. 2-10 to 2-12)	Kidney diseases (e.g., acute or chronic nephritis, nephritic syndrome); other (e.g., idiopathic edema)
Sunken qi (or failure of clear yang qi to rise)	Organ prolapse, abdominal distention, recurrent diarrhea or drooping eyelids (Figs. 2-17 and 2-18)	Prolapse of the stomach, kidney, rectum or uterus; diarrhea associated with chronic bowel disorders; myasthenia gravis
Dysfunction of the Spleen to govern the blood	Bleeding problems including some types of clotting disorders (Fig. 2-19)	Gastrointestinal hemorrhage (e.g., gastric or duodenal ulcer, ulcerative colitis); hematologic diseases (e.g., aplastic anemia, purpura [ITP]); menorrhagia (e.g., dysfunctional uterine bleeding [DUB]); other (hematuria, subcutaneous bleeding)
Spleen yang deficiency	Severe peripheral edema, or ascites with pale appearance and cold extremities (Figs. 2-13 and 2-14)	Edema, hydrothorax or hydroperitonium due to heart failure, kidney failure, chronic cor pulmonale, hepatic cirrhosis; malignant ascites
Tongue and pulse	Pale, swollen, and flabby tongue body with teeth marks around the border (Figs. 8-3 and 8-4); forceless pulse	

Acupuncture point selection principles:

Tonify the Spleen function and improve the qi activity

Selection of points:

BL-20, SP-3, CV-12, SP-6, ST-36, CV-6

Manipulation method:

Tonifying. If the case involves a combined pattern of deficiency and excess, the even movement or mild reducing method should be used.

Selection of points for complications:

- Excessive retention of dampness caused by Spleen deficiency: SP-9, ST-28, and KI-7
- Qi deficiency with stagnation: ST-21 and PC-6
- Poor digestion: CV-11 and SP-4

Table 2-2: *Acupuncture treatment*

Points	Explanation of Points	Combination of Points
BL-20	The organ-associated points of the back are very effective for tonifying the qi. BL-20 is used to tonify the Spleen.	These points relieve the symptoms caused by Spleen deficiency such as distention or pain in the abdomen, chest or intercostal regions, nausea or vomiting, constipation, or heaviness in the limbs or around the body.
SP-3	SP-3 is a source point of the Spleen channel which tonifies the Spleen, harmonizes the middle burner, and dispels dampness.	
CV-12	CV-12 is the alarm point of the Stomach. It is effective for harmonizing the middle burner.	The combination of CV-12 and SP-6 can be used for promoting qi activity and blood circulation, removing blood stasis, and regulating the functions of the middle and lower burners.
SP-6	SP-6 is the meeting point of the three yin foot channels and is used to nourish the lower burner (Kidney yin).	
ST-36	Tonifies the qi of the entire body and strengthens and harmonizes the middle burner.	ST-36 is closely related to the middle burner and CV-6 to the Kidney, both of which are important sources of qi. This two-point combination is commonly used to tonify the qi.
CV-6	As per its name, the "sea of qi," CV-6 is an excellent point for reinforcing the qi of the entire body.	

Treatment principle:

Tonify the qi and strengthen the Spleen.

Table 2-3: *Treatment with herbal formulas*

HERB AND DOSAGE	FLAVORS AND NATURE	ASSOCIATED CHANNELS	FORMULA ANALYSIS
■ Four-Gentlemen Decoction *(sì jūn zǐ tāng)* FOR TREATING DIFFERENT TYPES OF QI DEFICIENCY			
Ginseng Radix *(rén shēn),* 10g	Sweet and warm	Spleen and Lung	Tonifies the source qi of the entire body as well as the Spleen qi and Lung qi
Poria *(fú líng),* 9g	Sweet, bland, and neutral	Heart, Spleen, and Kidney	Tonify the qi and strengthen the Spleen, dry dampness, and relieve water metabolism disorder caused by qi deficiency
Atractylodis macrocephalae Rhizoma *(bái zhú),* 9g	Bitter, sweet, and warm	Spleen and Stomach	
Glycyrrhizae Radix *(gān cǎo),* 6g	Sweet and neutral	Heart, Lung, Spleen, and Stomach	Strengthens the Spleen and Stomach and protects the antipathogenic factors
■ Ginseng, Poria, and Atractylodes Macrocephala Powder *(shēn líng bái zhú sǎn)* FOR TREATING PATTERNS OF RETENTION OF DAMPNESS OR HARMFUL WATER CAUSED BY SPLEEN DEFICIENCY			
Ginseng Radix *(rén shēn),* 10g	Sweet and warm	Spleen and Lung	*Sì jūn zǐ tāng* is used in this formula to tonify the qi and strengthen the Spleen.
Poria *(fú líng),* 10g	Sweet, bland, and neutral	Heart, Spleen, and Kidney	
Atractylodis macrocephalae Rhizoma *(bái zhú),* 10g	Bitter, sweet, and warm	Spleen and Stomach	
Glycyrrhizae Radix *(gān cǎo),* 10g	Sweet and neutral	Heart, Lung, Spleen, and Stomach	

—*Continued next page*

HERB AND DOSAGE	FLAVORS AND NATURE	ASSOCIATED CHANNELS	FORMULA ANALYSIS
Dioscoreae Rhizoma *(shān yào)*, 10g	Sweet and neutral	Spleen, Lung, and Kidney	This group of herbs is used to strengthen the Spleen and promote the metabolism of water, thus draining dampness or pathogenic water from the body.
Lablab Semen album *(bái biăn dòu)*, 7.5g	Sweet and warm	Spleen and Stomach	
Coicis Semen *(yì yǐ rén)*, 5g	Sweet, bland, and slightly cold	Lung, Spleen, and Stomach	
Nelumbinis Semen *(lián zǐ)*, 5g	Sweet, astringent, and neutral	Spleen and Kidney	
Amomi Fructus *(shā rén)*, 5g	Acrid and warm	Spleen, Stomach, and Kidney	Dries dampness and regulates the qi
Platycodi Radix *(jié gěng)*, 5g	Bitter, acrid, and slightly warm	Lung	Benefits the Lung qi

■ Tonify the Middle to Augment the Qi Decoction *(bǔ zhōng yì qì tāng)*

FOR TREATING PROLAPSE OF THE ORGANS OR BLEEDING CAUSED BY PATTERNS OF QI DEFICIENCY

HERB AND DOSAGE	FLAVORS AND NATURE	ASSOCIATED CHANNELS	FORMULA ANALYSIS
Astragali Radix *(huáng qí)*, 15g	Sweet and warm	Spleen and Lung	Tonifies the qi and supports ascending action of the clear yang
Ginseng Radix *(rén shēn)*, 10g	Sweet and warm	Spleen and Lung	Four-Gentlemen Decoction *(sì jūn zǐ tāng)* is used to tonify the qi and strengthen the Spleen. Poria *(fú líng)* is omitted because no dampness exists here.
Atractylodis macrocephalae Rhizoma *(bái zhú)*, 10g	Bitter, sweet, and warm	Spleen and Stomach	
Glycyrrhizae Radix *(gān cǎo)*, 5g	Sweet and neutral	Heart, Lung, Spleen, and Stomach	
Citri reticulatae Pericarpium *(chén pí)*, 6g	Acrid, bitter, and warm	Spleen and Lung	Promotes the qi activity and strengthens the Spleen
Angelicae sinensis Radix *(dāng guī)*, 10g	Sweet, acrid, and warm	Liver and Heart	Nourishes the blood and dispels blood stasis
Cimicifugae Rhizoma *(shēng má)*, 3g	Sweet, acrid, and slightly cold	Lung, Spleen, and Stomach	Their rising characteristic supports the ascending action of the Spleen qi and clear yang and thus treats patterns of sinking qi (failure of clear yang qi to rise).
Bupleuri Radix *(chái hú)*, 3g	Bitter, acrid, and slightly cold	Liver and Gallbladder	

CHAPTER 3

Patterns of Blood Deficiency and Dual Qi and Blood Deficiency

Pale Mucous Membranes

Clinical manifestations

Pale membranes. Paleness can be seen at the inner lining of the eyelids (the conjunctivae), lips, inside the mouth, and in the tongue and nails.

Key points: See Figs. 3-1 through 3-4 (pp. 30-31).

Pathological process

The presence of pale membranes is an early and common sign of blood deficiency. The color of the mucous membranes, including the conjunctivae, reflects the local blood supply because the blood vessels run very close to the surface of the membranes and impart a pink hue to them. Because a change in the color of the mucous membranes reflects a change in blood flow in the vessels (viewed in Chinese medicine as an enrichment or deficiency of blood in the channels and collaterals), practitioners of both Western and Chinese medicine emphasize examination of the mucous membranes.

When there is blood deficiency there is a decrease of blood flowing through the channels and collaterals and therefore the conjunctivae and lips lose their normal color and appear pale.

In addition to changing the color of the mucous membranes, blood deficiency can also affect nourishment of the membranes, resulting in a loss of normal texture and moisture in the conjunctivae and lips, which thereupon appear dry, lifeless, and lacking in luster.

Diagnosis

Deficiency of blood or both blood and qi

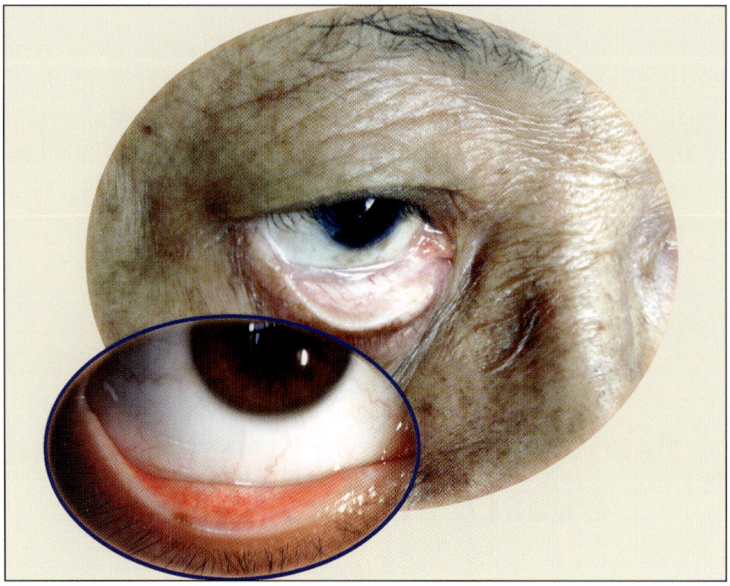

Fig. 3-1: *Anemia due to chronic renal failure*

Pale, dry, and lusterless conjunctivae with pale skin. The patient complains of slight discomfort in the eyes but no discharge or itchiness. (The small inset provides an example of normal-colored conjunctivae.)

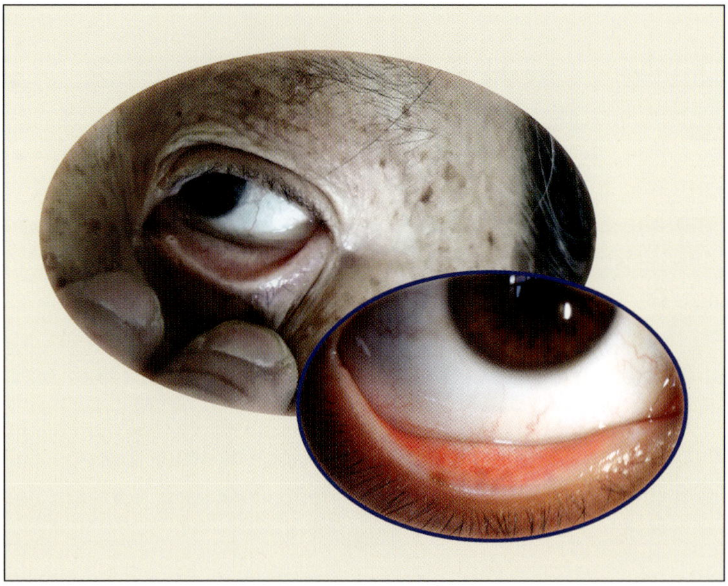

Fig. 3-2: *Iron deficiency anemia*

The complexion is sallow and lusterless and the conjunctivae have become lighter than normal. The insert picture shows a normal-colored conjunctiva lining the eyelids, which is pink, moist, and lustrous.

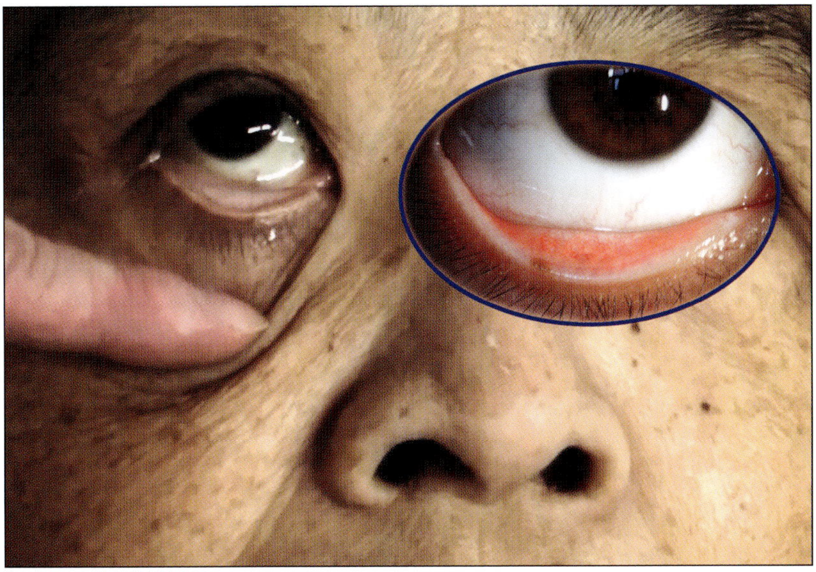

Fig. 3-3: *Hemolytic anemia with jaundice*

Significantly pale and lusterless conjunctivae. This patient is also shown in Fig. 6-21 in Chapter 6 on blood stasis.

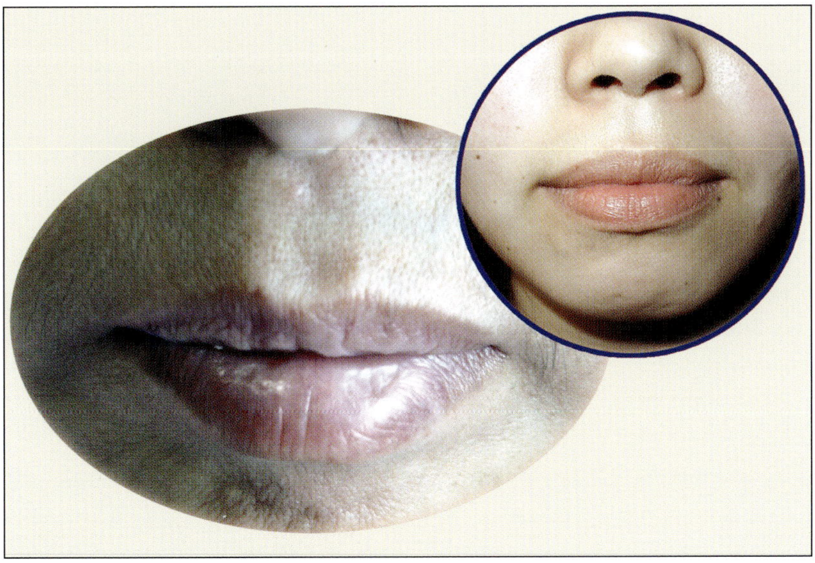

Fig. 3-4: *Kidney failure with uremia*

The lips are pale gray, dull, and lusterless. By way of comparison, see the insert picture of normal lips, which are pink, moist, lustrous, and have a fine texture.

Pale conjunctivae and lips indicate that the blood supply in the channels and collaterals is insufficient. Lusterless conjunctivae and shrivelled lips reflect malnourishment of blood in the mucous membranes.

Differential diagnosis

Anemia is frequently encountered in conventional Western medicine, and blood deficiency is a common pattern in Chinese medicine. The two conditions have many similarities in their symptoms and physical examination but should not be considered equivalent to one another.

When approaching a case of anemia, the signs and symptoms must be grouped into relevant categories in accordance with Chinese medical theory. Regarding the different types of anemia, iron deficiency anemia can be placed in the category of blood deficiency with Heart or Liver involvement; megaloblastic anemia (pernicious anemia) is more likely to be a pattern of dual qi and blood deficiency often involving the Heart and Spleen or the Spleen and Stomach; aplastic anemia and thalassemia may be placed in the pattern of qi or yang deficiency involving the Spleen and also the Kidney. Some patients with megaloblastic anemia may also fit into a pattern of qi and yin deficiency, which is complex and difficult to treat.

Abnormally Pale Skin

Clinical manifestations

Pale, lusterless, and dry skin

Key points: See Figs. 3-5 and 3-6 (p. 33).

Pathological process

Skin that has turned abnormally pale is another early and common sign of blood deficiency patterns. The skin color varies due to racial pigmentation. However, no matter what the skin tone, due to the blood in the collaterals a healthy skin color is a mixture of the basic color and a light rosy or pink hue. This indicates that the blood supply is normal and that there is sufficient yin and blood in the body.

Patients with blood deficiency do not have sufficient blood to supply the channels and collaterals and thus the skin color reflects this deficiency. This is most noticeable on the face. There is a classic saying in Chinese medicine that "the blood loses its ability to color the skin." The qi and yang of the body supply energy to circulate the blood, transport the water, and nourish the skin. When the qi becomes deficient, the skin also loses its normal color and becomes withered and pale; or it will be stretched and shiny with edema if yang deficiency is also present. (See Ch. 2 on qi deficiency for more details.)

Diagnosis

Blood deficiency or dual blood and qi deficiency

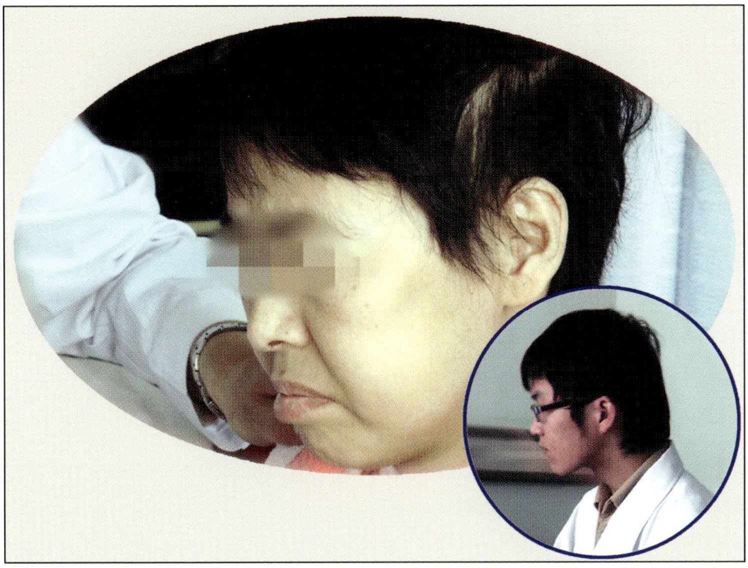

Fig. 3-5: *Kidney failure with uremia*

This is the same patient shown in Fig. 3-4. The patient has pale skin and looks weak and tired. By comparison, the doctor's complexion is shown in the insert. The lack of pink color in the skin of the patient is the most noticeable difference.

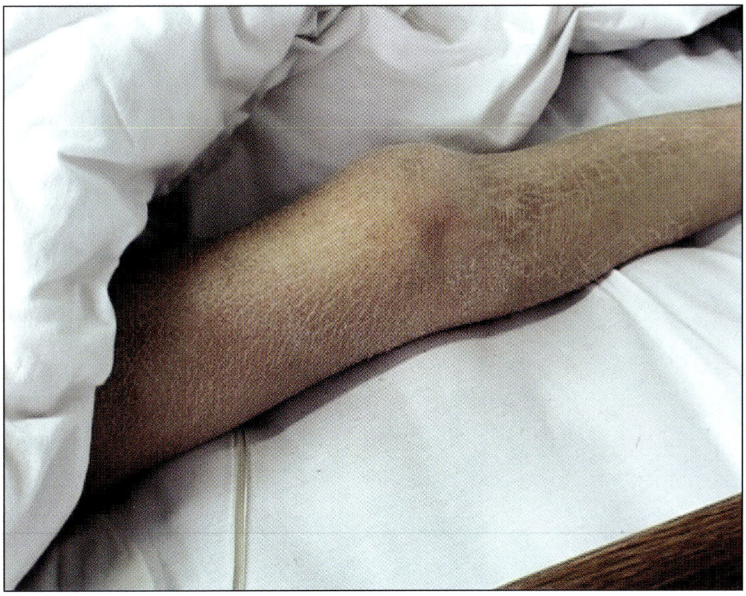

Fig. 3-6: *Subarachnoid hemorrhage (SAH) and loss of consciousness*

The skin of the lower extremities is dry, withered, and pale.

A pale complexion indicates a deficiency of blood. Withered and pale skin reflects a deficiency of qi as well as blood.

Differential diagnosis

A pale complexion is a basic characteristic of blood deficiency. Patterns of blood deficiency do not necessarily combine with yang deficiency, but if yang deficiency is present, the paleness of the complexion will be even more pronounced. Besides this change in the color of the complexion, the cardinal symptoms for determining the existence of yang deficiency are associated with cold, such as intolerance of cold and cold extremities.

Withered and Sallow Skin

Clinical manifestations

A sallow, dull, and lusterless complexion that may be accompanied by wrinkles, flabby and withered skin, or reduced skin turgor (elasticity)

Key points: See Figs. 3-7 though 3-9 (pp. 35-36).

Pathological process

Sallow and withered skin or decreased skin turgor (elasticity) are clinical manifestations of the skin's loss of normal nourishment.

As previously noted, the color and general appearance of the skin are different aspects in the examination of the complexion. No matter what the color, a healthy appearance of the skin refers to luster (or brightness), good skin turgor, and bloom, the presence of which implies that there is a sufficient supply of blood and qi to the skin.

A deficiency of blood means that there will be an insufficient supply reaching the surface of the body. As a result, a patient's normal complexion will change and become either pale, as shown in Figs. 3-5 and 3-6, or sallow and lusterless, as shown in Figs. 3-7 to 3-9.

A deficiency of qi, especially Spleen qi, may impair the skin's ability to derive nourishment from the essence of food and body fluids. The luster thus disappears and the skin becomes darker and more sallow. Reduced skin turgor causes wrinkles to appear on the surface as well as flabby, withered skin. (See Ch. 2 on Spleen qi deficiency for more details.)

Diagnosis

A pattern of dual blood and qi deficiency

The normal rosy color of the skin becomes pale or completely disappears, indicating a deficiency of blood. The skin becomes sallow or sallow and withered, indicating that a deficiency of qi is also present.

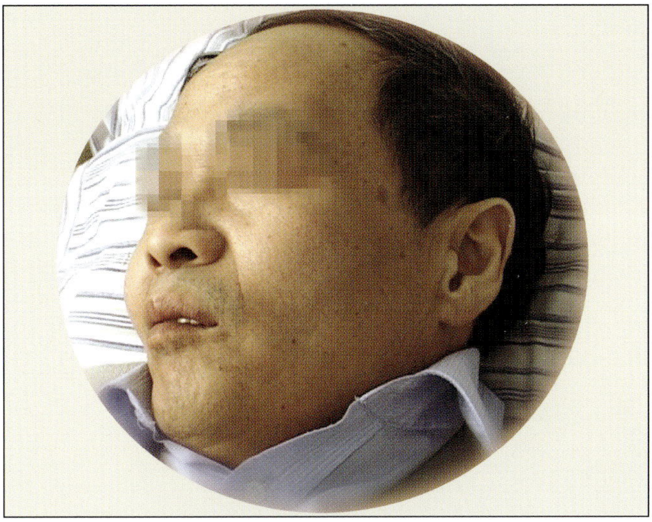

Fig. 3-7: *Iron deficiency anemia*

The complexion is sallow and lusterless, and the normal rosy color of the face has disappeared.

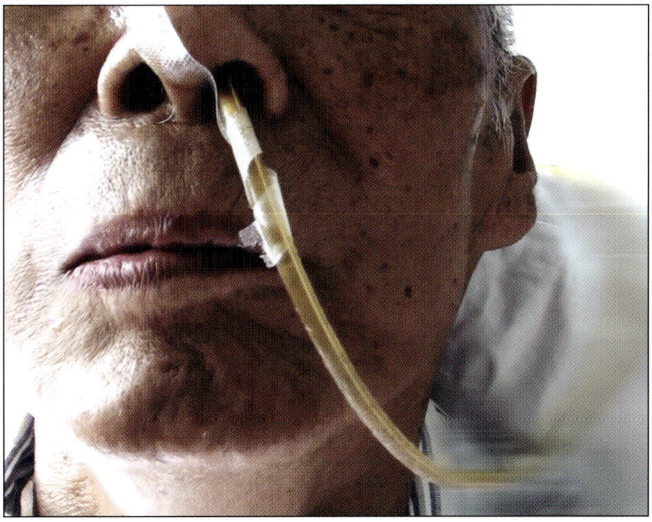

Fig. 3-8: *Ischemic stroke*

The complexion is withered, noticeably sallow, and the skin tone is poor.

Differential diagnosis

Depending on the individual's race, human skin color can range from very dark to very fair. However, regardless of race, normal skin tone should have a healthy bloom and luster. Thus a complexion in which the basic skin tone has bloom and luster is considered to be normal.

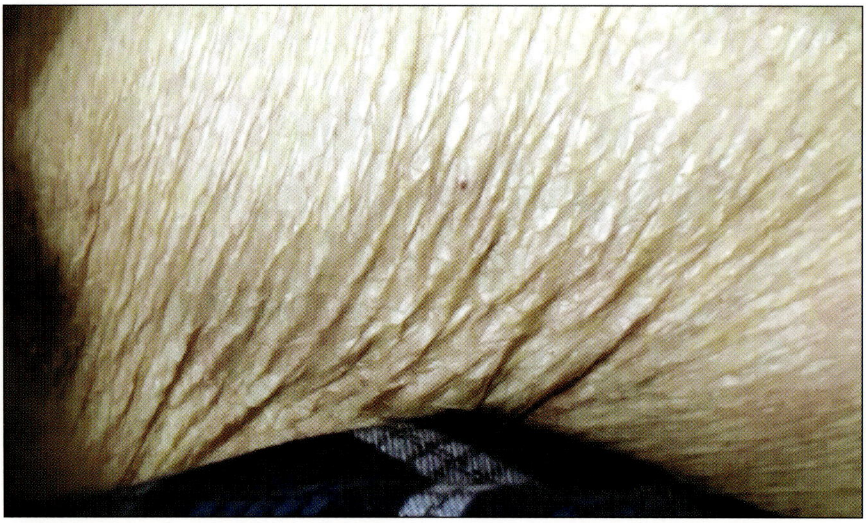

Fig. 3-9: *Advanced stage of cirrhosis*
The skin on the trunk is lusterless, flabby, and withered, and has very poor skin turgor.

In those with light or medium brown skin, such as people of Asian descent, paleness is associated with blood deficiency while sallow and withered skin indicates a pattern of dual qi and blood deficiency, especially when this pattern is caused by a deficiency of Spleen qi.

For those with lighter skin, such as people of European descent, a deficiency of blood itself results in the normal rosiness becoming pale, as the blood fails to color the skin. When there is a dual deficiency of qi and blood, the skin becomes withered and more pale, but not sallow. That is to say, in light or "white" skin, the paleness is prominent but the sallowness may be masked.

For those with darker skin, such as people of African descent, a deficiency of blood itself results in the complexion losing its bloom. When there is a dual deficiency of qi and blood, the skin appears even darker than normal and its lack of luster becomes much more obvious, but it does not become pale or sallow. That is to say, in a dark-skinned person, the lack of luster is prominent but the paleness or sallowness may be difficult to discern.

Muscle Spasms or Cramps

Clinical manifestations

Numbness in the limbs, an abnormal increase in muscle tension (hypertonia), muscle spasticity or cramps, or contraction of the joints

Key points: See Figs. 3-10 and 3-11 (p. 37).

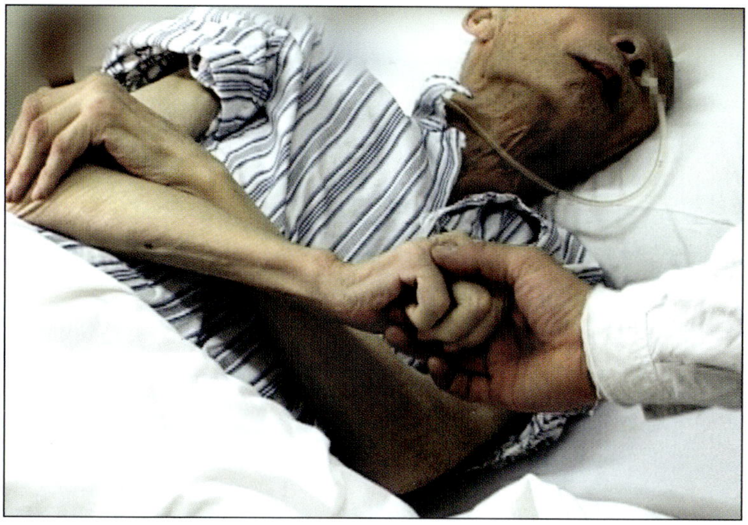

Fig. 3-10: *Cerebrovascular disease (ischemic stroke) with unconsciousness*

Emaciated limbs with wrinkled, withered, and sallow skin. This image shows a spastic hypertonia involving muscle spasticity of arms and clenched fingers.

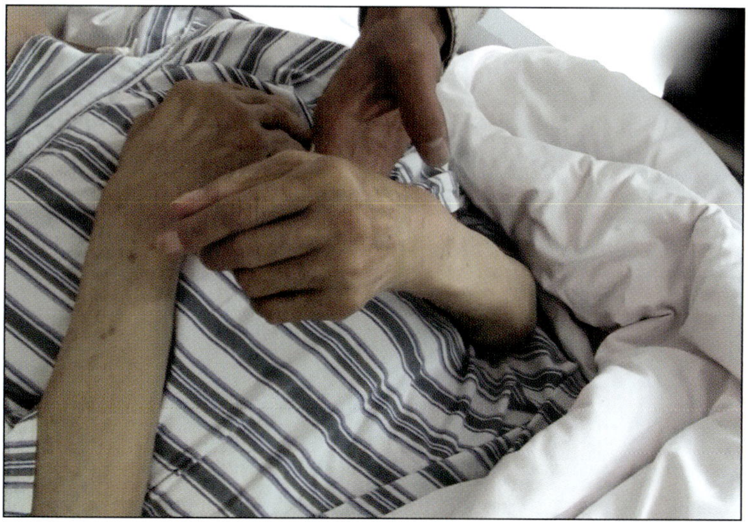

Fig. 3-11: *The reduced ability of a muscle to stretch*

This image shows a patient with bent elbows and muscle resistance to passive stretching. After passive stretching, his arms return to an involuntary fixed position.

Pathological process

Inflexibility and stiffness in the limbs resulting from an abnormal and prolonged contraction of the ligaments and tendons (or sinews)

An important function of the Liver is to store blood, thus Chinese medicine refers to the Liver as the "sea of blood." Additionally, the Liver is the organ that controls the ligaments and tendons (sinews). This means that the ligaments and tendons are nourished by the Liver blood, thus facilitating movement of the muscles.

A deficiency of blood implies an insufficiency of Liver blood. When the sea of blood is insufficient, the undernourished ligaments and tendons lose their ability to control the flexibility and agility of the joints and thus spasms and cramps can occur. In this particular case, the elbows are bent and the fingers clenched. Long-term illness can severely consume the yin (or essence) and yang qi in the body, here marked by emaciated limbs with sallow, wrinkled, and withered skin.

Diagnosis

Blood and qi deficiency along with internal wind caused by deficiency of blood

Emaciated limbs associated with sallow, wrinkled, and withered skin indicate that both the qi and blood are deficient. The increase in muscle tension and diminished ability of a muscle to stretch, muscle spasticity, and arms fixed in an involuntary position all indicate a deficiency of blood resulting in malnourishment of the ligaments and tendons.

Differential diagnosis

Symptoms such as muscle cramps or spasms, tetany (as seen in hypocalcemia), shaking, convulsions or seizure, muscle twitching or fasciculation and hemiplegia, bent fingers or elbows are all called *dòng fēng* (动风) in Chinese medicine, meaning "stirred-up wind." The wind referred to is internal wind. There are four different causes of internal wind:

- A preponderance of Liver yang (or ascendant Liver yang) results in a wind pattern.
- Extreme heat leads to wind.
- Interior wind is caused by blood deficiency.
- Interior wind is caused by yin deficiency.

In this case, the wind is caused by blood deficiency and the key points for diagnosis are the symptoms of blood deficiency and the muscle cramps or spasms.

Dry, Itchy, or Cracked Skin

Clinical manifestations

The skin loses its moisture and becomes dry and itchy, or it may become rough, thick, and cracked. The problem can be either local or generalized.

Key points: See Figs. 3-12 and 3-13 (p. 39).

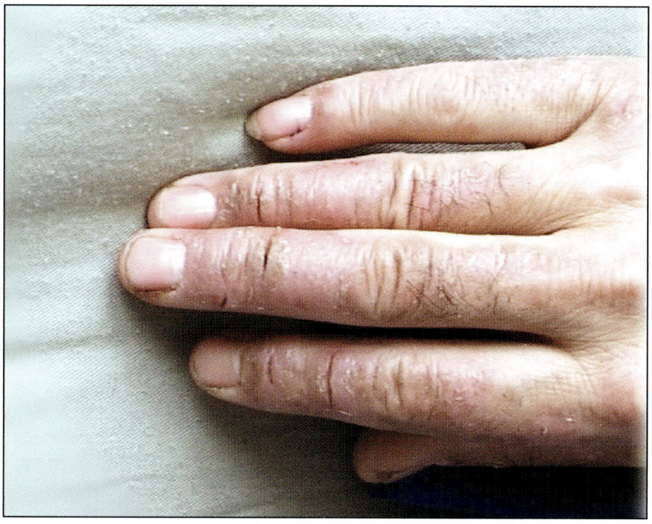

Fig. 3-12: *Atopic dermatitis*

Dry, lusterless, and brittle skin; scales can be seen on the fingers. Thickened skin and a greater depth in the lines in the skin cause it to take on a leathery texture or lichenification. The fissures are quite prominent, giving a cracked appearance to the skin of the fingers.

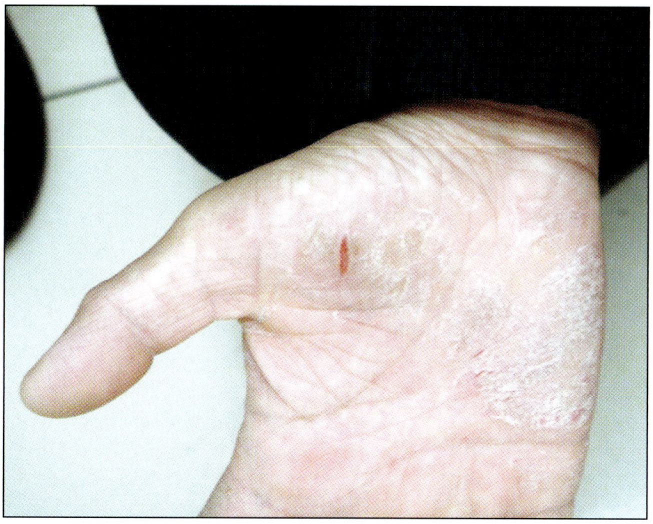

Fig. 3-13: *Another case of atopic dermatitis*
Thickened skin and fissures on the palm

Pathological process

Dry, itchy, and brittle skin is the result of malnourishment of the skin due to a deficiency of blood.

Blood, especially the fluid portion of the blood, plays an important function in maintaining an optimum level of moisture in the body, including proper moisturizing of the skin. In the case of blood deficiency, reduced hydration in the body gives rise to symptoms characterized by dryness. This pathological process is referred to as a pattern of interior dryness.

As dryness leads to dehydration of the body and insufficient hydration of the skin, the skin becomes dry, lusterless, and scaly. The fingers are most affected, as they are located at the extremities and receive the least moisturization.

The appearance of leathery skin also indicates a pattern of interior dryness caused by blood deficiency. Internal dryness causes the skin to become itchy and brittle and to lose its flexibility. Chronic and repeated scratching can worsen thickened skin (lichenification). The rough and thickened skin is less elastic and the depth of the skin lines increases; this aggravates the dehydration of the skin and affects areas where the skin creases, so that it begins to crack and bleed.

Diagnosis

Interior dryness caused by blood deficiency

Scaly, dry, and itchy skin indicates that the cause of the problem is pathogenic dryness. Thick, cracked skin and lichenification indicate a deficiency of blood resulting in a dry pattern.

Differential diagnosis

The cause of dry, or dry and itchy skin (xerosis) can be due to either an internal or external pathogenic factor.

The external pathogenic factors in the environment that cause skin conditions are pathogenic cold or dryness. These factors often occur during the dry seasons of fall or winter. On the other hand, an internal pathogenic factor that causes such conditions is internal dryness, which often results from patterns like heat consuming the body fluids (detailed in Ch. 5, and shown in Figs. 3-8 and 3-9), blood deficiency or yin deficiency, described in this section.

The difference between external and internal dryness is that external dryness is closely associated with seasonal changes and its symptoms tend to be mild, and even gradually disappear, as the seasons change. By contrast, internal dryness is more severe, the disease can last much longer, and, as internal dryness has no connection with the environment, a change of season will offer no significant improvement.

Loss of Hair

Clinical manifestations

Localized hair loss which causes completely bald areas, or generalized hair loss and a diffuse thinning of hair. The hair looks dull, lusterless, and dry, or the hair is brittle and is broken easily or split at the ends.

Key points: See Figs. 3-14 and 3-15 below.

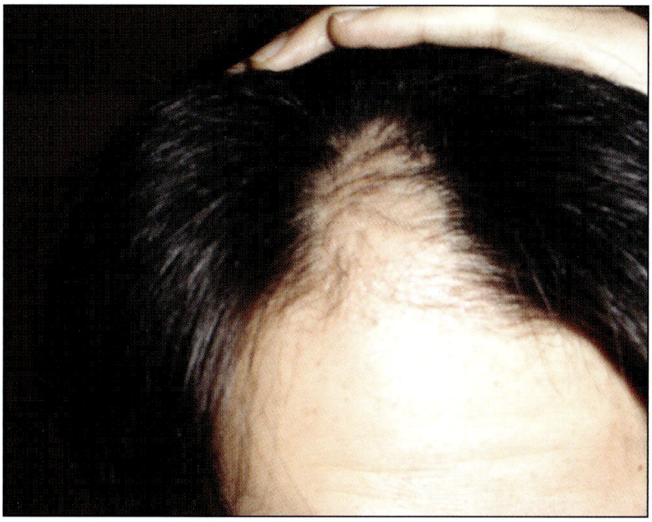

Fig. 3-14: *Alopecia areata*

A patch of sudden hair loss. There is a clear boundary between the normal hair and the area affected by alopecia.

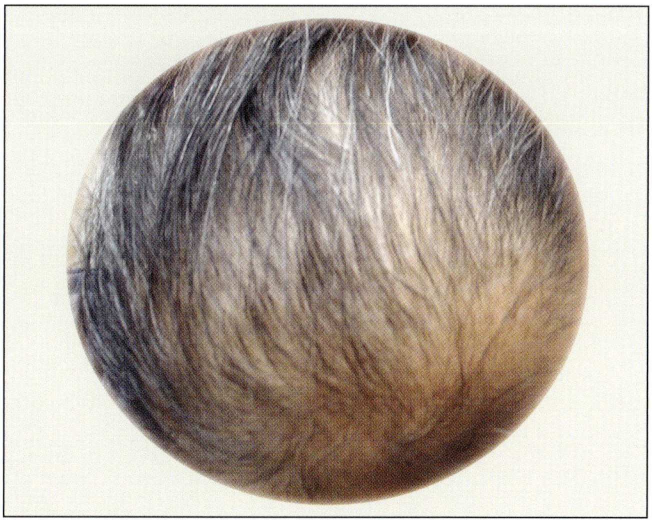

Fig. 3-15: *Another patient with excessive hair loss*

Thin, dull, lusterless hair. This is diffuse hair loss affecting large areas of the scalp.

Pathological process

The hair has lost the nutrition supplied it by the blood.

In Chinese medical theory the hair reflects the surplus of blood. A sufficient supply of blood is essential for the growth and healthy appearance of the hair. Blood deficiency or poor circulation in the scalp can result in a loss of normal nutrition to the hair, leading to a diffuse thinning of the hair.

Malnutrition of the hair means a reduction in or absence of the essence needed to maintain the hair's normal sheen and texture, such that it loses its luster and suppleness, becoming dull and dry, easily broken, or split at the ends.

Patches of hair loss (alopecia areata) is a special subtype of hair loss caused by blood deficiency in which pathogenic factors strangle the circulation to the scalp. A patient with blood deficiency (either blood deficiency in a specific area that is part of general blood deficiency in the body, or due to something directly causing a small area to have blood deficiency) can be attacked by pathogenic factors (e.g., external pathogenic wind) or emotional stress. Blocked collaterals deplete the nourishment to local surfaces of the scalp, and thus alopecia is the direct result.

Diagnosis

Deficiency of blood or deficiency of blood and invasion by pathogenic wind

Both diffuse, thinning hair which is dull, lusterless, and dry as well as patches of hair loss indicate a pattern of blood deficiency. Sudden onset of the condition indicates that the patient has suffered an invasion by pathogenic wind. A clear boundary between the patch of hair loss and the normal hair indicates that the site of the disease is superficial and that the pathogenic factors only block the superficial collaterals.

Differential diagnosis

Excessive hair loss can be diagnosed as either deficient or excessive.

Practitioners should note that these two types of patterns have different manifestations. Generalized hair loss (such as female pattern baldness, or hair loss associated with systemic diseases) and patchy hair loss (such as alopecia areata) are commonly caused by blood deficiency or Kidney deficiency.

Excessive patterns (such as alopecia due to seborrheic dermatitis of the scalp) are caused by heat in the blood (see Ch. 4, which addresses hot blood, for more details). Because the pathological processes are different, the patterns are different and thus the treatments are quite opposite each other. A common mistake in clinical practice is to fail to distinguish the two disorders and to simply nourish the blood in order to treat both, which is wrong.

Pale Tongue

When there are patterns of blood deficiency or qi and blood dual deficiency, the tongue becomes paler. (See Ch. 8, which deals with tongue diagnosis, for more details.)

Summary

Table 3.1: *Key diagnostic points for patterns of blood deficiency and dual qi and blood deficiency*

Cause	Symptoms (Images)	Examples of Diseases and Symptoms
Blood loses its ability to color the skin and membranes	Pale and lusterless eyelids, lips, tongue, nails and skin, or withered and sallow skin (Figs. 3-1 to 3-9)	Anemia (e.g., iron deficiency anemia), blood loss (e.g., childbirth, injury or surgery), malnutrition (e.g., post-gastrectomy malabsorption); chronic conditions (e.g., cancers, infection)
Malnourishment of the organs	Dizziness, blurred vision, palpitations, poor memory, insomnia or excessive dreaming	Cardiovascular disease (e.g., arrhythmia), autonomic nervous system disorders (e.g., orthostatic hypotension); other: insomnia, neurosis, anxiety, or depression
Internal wind caused by blood deficiency	Numbness in hands, feet, or other parts of the body	Cerebrovascular diseases (e.g., transient ischemic attack), abnormal sensation caused by neurological disorders (e.g., paresthesia or hyperesthesia)
	Muscle spasms or cramps, inflexibility of the limbs (Figs. 3-10 and 3-11)	Cerebrovascular diseases (e.g., stroke), electrolyte abnormalities (e.g., hypocalcemia), neuromuscular disorder (e.g., multiple sclerosis)
Malnutrition of hair caused by blood deficiency	Localized or generalized hair loss (Figs. 3-14 and 3-15)	Hair loss: alopecia areata or alopecia totalis, female-pattern baldness, hair loss associated with systemic diseases
Skin loses moisture resulting from blood deficiency	Dryness of the skin, eyes, mouth, or nose (Figs. 3-12 and 3-13)	Skin conditions (e.g., chronic eczema, xerosis), autoimmune (e.g., Sjogren's syndrome); other: side effects of radiation or chemotherapy
Deficiency of the sea of blood (Penetrating vessel)	Delayed menstruation, irregular or missed menstrual cycle, flow with pinkish color	Menstrual problems (e.g., scanty menses, secondary amenorrhea)
Dual qi and blood deficiency	Pale or sallow and lusterless skin with such symptoms as fatigue, weakness, lack of energy, shortness of breath or emaciation (Figs. 3-1 to 3-9)	Anemia (e.g., pernicious anemia), chronic disease (e.g., infections, cancers), recovery from diseases or surgery, neuromuscular disorder (e.g., multiple sclerosis)
Tongue and pulse	Pale tongue body, thin pulse (Figs. 8-1 and 8-2)	

Acupuncture point selection principles:

Nourish the blood and tonify the qi because qi and blood depend on each other and transform into each other. The Spleen qi is responsible for producing blood.

Selection of points:

BL-17, SP-6, CV-17, CV-12, CV-6, LU-9, ST-36

Manipulation method:

Reinforcing method

Selection of points for complications:

- Dizziness and blurred vision: GB-20
- Insomnia and poor memory: HT-7, M-HN-1
- Numbness of the extremities or muscle spasms: LI-10, GB-34
- Prolonged period: KI-13

Table 3-2: *Acupuncture treatment*

Points	Point Explanation	Point Combination
BL-17	The influential point of the blood, it is very effective for nourishing the yin and blood.	The combination of both points can be used to nourish the yin and blood.
SP-6	The meeting point of the three yin foot channels, it has the general effect of nourishing the blood.	
CV-17	As an influential point of the qi, CV-17 is used for regulating the directional flow of qi throughout the body.	These points promote the function of the Triple Burner, regulate qi activities, and remove obstruction from the channels and collaterals.
CV-12	The alarm point of the Stomach, it is used to regulate the qi in the middle burner.	
CV-6	One of the most important points for treating disorders of qi and/or blood. It can reinforce and regulate the qi and also harmonize the blood.	
LU-9	The source point of the hand greater yin channel and the influential point for the blood vessels, it is thus a good point to regulate both the qi and blood.	These are the supporting points for CV-17, CV-12, and CV-6. They promote qi to strengthen the source of the production of blood.
ST-36	A very important tonifying point. By strengthening the function of the middle burner, a healthy Spleen will support the generation of blood.	

Treatment principles:

Nourish the blood, or tonify the qi and nourish the blood

Table 3-3: *Treatment with herbal formulas*

HERB AND DOSAGE	FLAVORS AND NATURE	ASSOCIATED CHANNELS	FORMULA ANALYSIS

■ Four-Substance Decoction *(sì wù tāng)*

BASIC FORMULA FOR NOURISHING THE BLOOD

HERB AND DOSAGE	FLAVORS AND NATURE	ASSOCIATED CHANNELS	FORMULA ANALYSIS
Rehmanniae Radix preparata *(shú dì huáng)*, 12g	Sweet and slightly warm	Heart, Liver, and Kidney	Nourishes the blood and yin
Angelicae sinensis Radix *(dāng guī)*, 10g	Sweet , acrid, and warm	Liver and Heart	Nourishes the blood and dispels blood stasis; also good for alleviating pain and regulating periods
Chuanxiong Rhizoma *(chuān xiōng)*, 8g	Acrid and warm	Liver and Gallbladder	Removes blood stasis and improves the circulation of qi
Paeoniae Radix alba *(bái sháo)*, 12g	Sour and cold	Liver and Spleen	Nourishes the blood and yin

■ Emperor of Heaven's Special Pill to Tonify the Heart *(tiān wáng bǔ xīn dān)*

FOR NOURISHING THE BLOOD AND CALMING THE SPIRIT

HERB AND DOSAGE	FLAVORS AND NATURE	ASSOCIATED CHANNELS	FORMULA ANALYSIS
Rehmanniae Radix *(shēng dì huáng)*, 24g	Sweet, bitter, and cold	Heart, Liver, and Kidney	Nourishes the yin and blood
Angelicae sinensis Radix *(dāng guī)*, 12g	Sweet, acrid, and warm	Liver and Heart	Nourish the blood
Salviae miltiorrhizae Radix *(dān shēn)*, 6g	Bitter and slightly cold	Liver and Heart	
Scrophulariae Radix *(xuán shēn)*, 6g	Bitter, salty, and cold	Lung, Stomach, and Kidney	Nourish the yin
Asparagi Radix *(tiān mén dōng)*, 12g	Sweet, bitter, and cold	Lung and Kidney	
Ophiopogonis Radix *(mài mén dōng)*, 12g	Sweet and cold	Lung, Heart, and Stomach	

—*continued next page*

HERB AND DOSAGE	FLAVORS AND NATURE	ASSOCIATED CHANNELS	FORMULA ANALYSIS
Ginseng Radix *(rén shēn)*, 6g	Sweet and warm	Spleen and Lung	Tonify the qi and strengthen the Spleen
Poria *(fú líng)*, 6g	Sweet, bland, and neutral	Heart, Spleen, and Kidney	
Polygalae Radix *(yuǎn zhì)*, 6g	Bitter, acrid, and warm	Heart and Lung	Tonify the Heart and calm the spirit
Ziziphi spinosae Semen *(suān zǎo rén)*, 12g	Sweet and neutral	Heart, Liver, and Gallbladder	
Platycladi Semen *(bǎi zǐ rén)*, 12g	Sweet and neutral	Heart	
Schisandrae Fructus *(wǔ wèi zǐ)*, 6g	Sour and warm	Lung, Kidney, and Heart	
Platycodi Radix *(jié gěng)*, 6g	Bitter, acrid, and slightly warm	Lung	Benefits the Lung qi

■ **Eight-Treasure Decoction** *(bā zhēn tāng)*

FOR TREATING PATTERNS OF DUAL QI AND BLOOD DEFICIENCY

Ginseng Radix *(rén shēn)*, 3g	Sweet and warm	Spleen and Lung	Four-Gentlemen Decoction *(sì jūn zǐ tāng)* tonifies the qi
Poria *(fú líng)*, 8g	Sweet, bland, and neutral	Heart, Spleen, and Kidney	
Atractylodis macrocephalae Rhizoma *(bái zhú)*, 10g	Bitter, sweet, and warm	Spleen and Stomach	
Glycyrrhizae Radix *(gān cǎo)*, 5g	Sweet and neutral	Heart, Lung, Spleen, and Stomach	
Rehmanniae Radix preparata *(shú dì huáng)*, 15g	Sweet and slightly warm	Heart, Liver, and Kidney	Four-Substance Decoction *(sì wù tāng)* nourishes the blood
Angelicae sinensis Radix *(dāng guī)*, 10g	Sweet, acrid, and warm	Liver and Heart	
Chuanxiong Rhizoma *(chuān xiōng)*, 5g	Acrid and warm	Liver and Gallbladder	
Paeoniae Radix alba *(bái sháo)*, 8g	Sour and cold	Liver and Spleen	

CHAPTER 4

Patterns of Hot Blood

Red Skin

Clinical manifestations

Skin lesions with scales affecting different parts of the body

Key points: See Figs. 4-1 through 4-3 (pp. 48-49).

Pathological process

Red skin is a common and early symptom of hot blood patterns.

Heat is a yang pathogenic factor characterized by a tendency to force itself outward. When heat accelerates the circulation of the blood, it causes concentration of blood in the soft tissue close to the skin surface (the interstices and pores), which explains why the skin is red.

Furthermore, blood is part of the yin of the body, which nourishes the skin. As heat causes the fluid in the blood to evaporate, it consumes the nutrient yin, interfering with its function of nourishing and moisturizing the skin. The skin thus becomes dry, and flakes—which are readily shed—appear.

Diagnosis

Hot blood pattern with pathogenic heat in the blood, accompanied by a dry pattern caused by hot blood (the result of evaporation of the body fluids and yin due to heat).

Scattered skin lesions on the trunk or extremities indicate that the pathogenic factors in the body are not yet serious. Red skin lesions are evidence of heat patterns. Lesions covered by scales indicate a dry pattern caused by hot blood. The heat has consumed the yin and body fluids and has caused dryness of the skin.

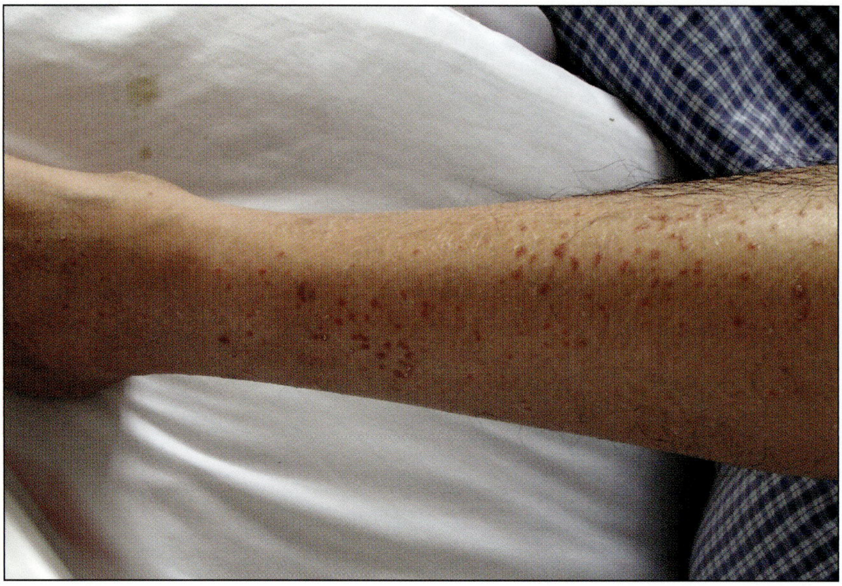

Fig. 4-1: *Psoriasis*

New-onset psoriatic skin lesions. Generalized small erythematous, guttate papules with mild scales have appeared on the patient's extremities.

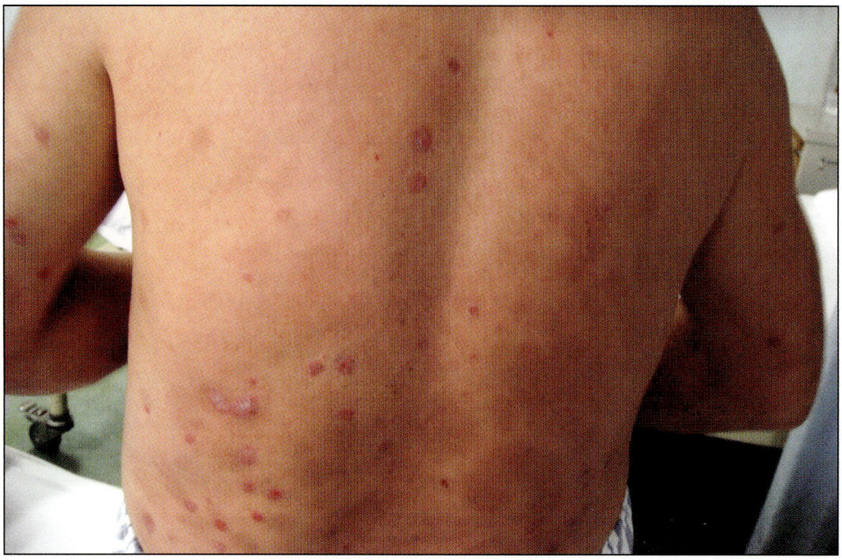

Fig. 4-2: *Another case of psoriasis*

Red, pruritic papules and plaques have developed over the trunk.

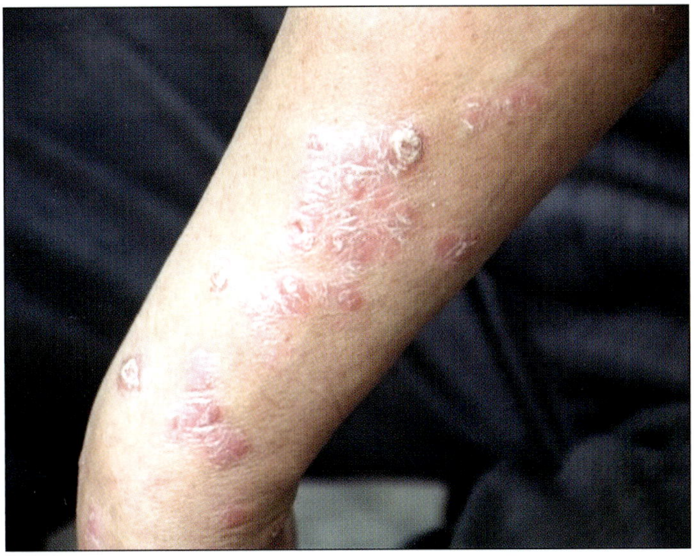

Fig. 4-3: *Close-up of psoriatic skin lesions*
The skin lesions are dry, thick, and crusty, and have white or silvery scales that easily fall off.

Differential diagnosis

In clinical practice there are two different types of dry patterns: exterior and interior.

Exterior dry patterns typically include a history of an invasion of external dryness from the exterior, symptoms of dryness, and the general symptoms of exterior patterns.

Interior dryness, on the other hand, is associated with blood or yin deficiency (detailed in Ch. 3 on blood deficiency) or may emerge as a deficiency of body fluids resulting from heat consumption, as in this case. Besides dryness of the skin, the symptoms of these patterns are associated with a deficiency of general body fluids, but without any symptoms of an exterior pattern.

Widespread Red Skin

Clinical manifestations

Large areas of red, thick, and dry skin

Key points: See Figs. 4-4 through 4-6 (pp. 50-51).

Pathological process

In this group of images, the affected area of skin is much more widespread compared with the case shown above (Figs. 4-1 through 4-3).

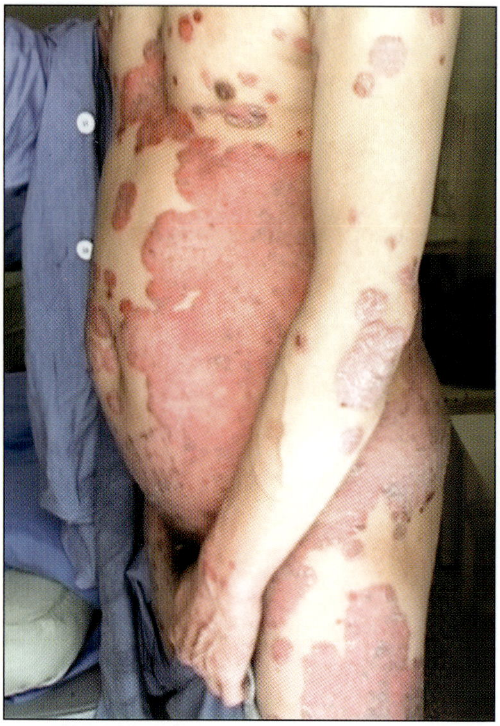

Fig. 4-4: *Psoriasis*

The image shows generalized plaques (reddish areas of thickened skin) that have merged, producing a large confluent erythma on the body.

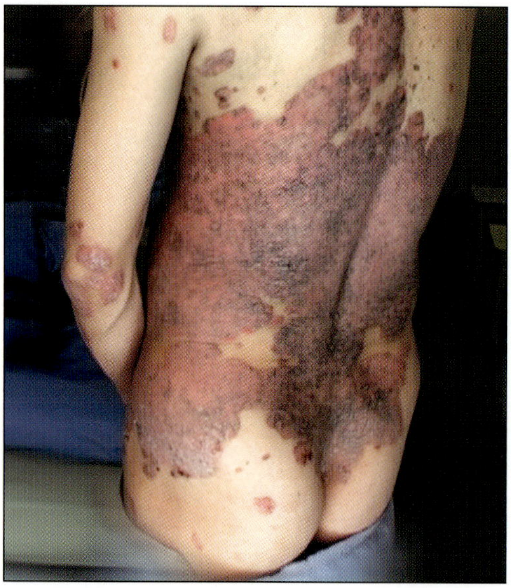

Fig. 4-5: *Same patient shown above*

Extensive red plaques with scales cover large areas of his body. The affected skin is coarse and thick.

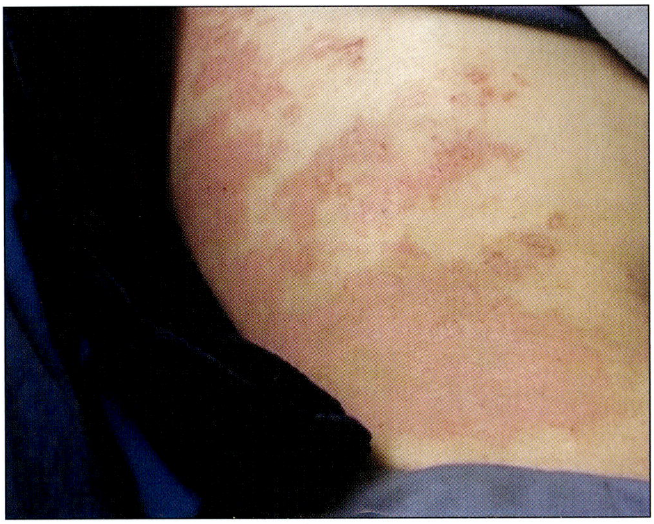

Fig. 4-6: *Eczema*

Red rashes cover most of the body.

Plaques occurring on the skin are a result of blood accumulating in the skin surface (the "interstices and pores" of the skin, as it is known in Chinese medicine), caused by heat accelerating the circulation of blood.

When blood circulates in the channels and collaterals, it can spread pathogenic heat outward and around the entire body, causing the plaques on the skin to join together and produce a large, confluent, erythematous plaque covering much of the body. The heat evaporates the body fluids and consumes the blood, thus leading to malnourishment of the skin, which thereupon becomes thick, crusty, and covered in scales.

Diagnosis

Hot blood pattern with excessive heat existing in the blood level

Red plaques indicate heat in the blood. Thick, coarse, and crusty skin covered in scales indicates malnourishment of the skin. Plaques joining together to create large plaques reflect a severe and progressive stage of the disorder.

In the case shown in Fig. 4-6, the heat in the blood is relatively mild compared with that shown in Figs. 4-4 and 4-5.

Differential diagnosis

In modern medicine, this group of images represents two different conditions—psoriasis and eczema—but according to the basic theory and diagnostic method of Chinese medicine, both cases belong to hot blood patterns.

Traditional Chinese medicine differentiates between two levels of hot blood patterns: a nutritive level and a blood level. (This distinction will be discussed below in connection with rashes.) The blood level pattern is further subdivided into two types: the excessive aspect of heat in the blood level and the deficient aspect of heat in the blood level. The key point for differentiating these two subtypes is to determine whether strong heat is present in the blood.

If heat—reflected in a high body temperature, large plaques on the skin, and hemorrhaging in severe cases—is the main symptom, then an excessive type is evident. If the heat is from deficiency, or there is empty heat in the blood level, with such symptoms as tidal heat (afternoon heat) becoming dominant, then a deficient type is present.

Widespread Bright Red Skin

Clinical manifestations

Widespread bright red skin affects most of the body surface. The skin becomes hot and dry.

Key points: See Figs. 4-7 and 4-8 (p. 53).

Pathological process

The distinctive feature in this case is severe and widespread pathogenic heat.

When pathogenic heat in the blood develops to an extreme level, it evolves into heat toxin. This toxin follows the blood in its circulation around the entire body and causes the bright red coloration of the skin, which almost loses its normal appearance.

The pathogenic heat disperses through the skin and thus the skin is hot to the touch.

Swelling around the elbows is due to increased blood flow to the collaterals on the outer surface of the body.

Since the onset of the condition is acute with a short history, no serious damage has been done to the body's blood and yin. Therefore scaling of the skin only appears on the arms and there is no significant coarsening or thickening of the skin on the trunk. This suggests that the heat in the blood is quite strong but that the skin is not yet severely malnourished.

Diagnosis

Hot blood pattern, with strong pathogenic heat in the blood

This is a severe pattern of excessive heat in the blood level. The bright red skin which is hot to the touch indicates extreme heat in the blood. The swollen limbs indicate an accumulation and stagnation of qi and blood in the channels and collaterals. Pathogenic heat has already spread out over the entire body and therefore most of the skin is affected, indicating that the condition has reached a severe stage.

Differential diagnosis

Among the cases presented so far, this patient (Figs. 4-7 and 4-8) has the most severe

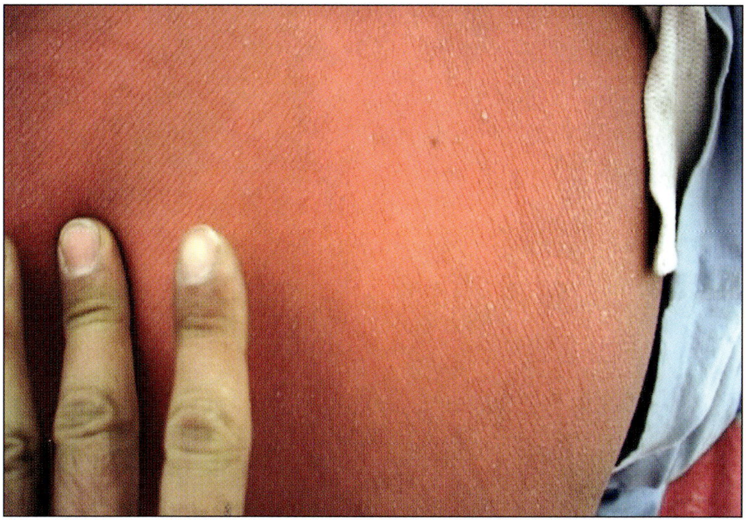

Fig. 4-7: *Erythrodermic psoriasis (psoriasic erythroderma)*
Large areas of the skin are fiery red and dry. The body is hot to the touch. The skin on the back appears smooth, with a normal texture. There are no apparent scales on the trunk.

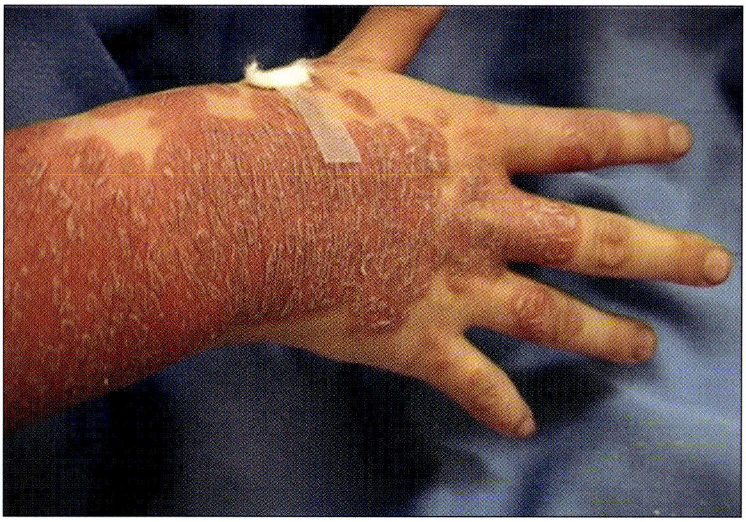

Fig. 4-8: *Reddening and scaling of the skin on the forearms*
Swelling (edema) around the wrists has also developed.

pathogenic heat. Clinically, erythroderma is a symptom seen with different causes, for example, in psoriasis, eczema, or drug rashes. Although these are different conditions in conventional medicine, in Chinese medicine the diagnosis and treatment of erythroderma of any type are similar irrespective of the cause, because of the similarity of the symptoms and pathological processes.

Red, Dry, and Itchy Skin

Clinical manifestations

Itchy and red skin with fever and irritability. Measles-like rashes or red, raised, and irregularly shaped patches may appear on the skin. Scaly skin can be observed in some patients.

Key points: See Figs. 4-9 and 4-10 (p. 55).

Pathological process

Itchy skin with reduced elasticity indicates the presence of internal wind and a deficiency of body fluids (patterns of dryness).

In Chinese medicine, itchy skin (pruritus) is often associated with special types of patterns called wind-dryness caused by hot blood (*xuè rè fēng zào zhèng* 血热风燥证). In these patterns, heat in the blood results in dryness, which stirs up internal wind. The pathological process is that blood, one of the body fluids, has a yin nature with the functions of moisturizing and nourishing the skin to prevent dryness. The presence of pathogenic heat can evaporate and exhaust the fluids in the blood, resulting in patterns of internal dryness. If the dryness develops further, it may generate internal wind. Itchy skin then ensues as the internal wind disturbs the harmony between nutritive yin (blood) and protective yang (qi) in the skin (the "interstices and pores").

This pathological process of itching, according to Chinese medical theory, is similar to what occurs in nature: severe heat in a desert results in a lack of moisture in the air, which causes dry, windy air. Chinese medicine compares this natural phenomenon to the pathological process associated with the human body and calls this a pattern of wind-dryness caused by hot blood.

Pathogenic heat stimulates the circulation of blood, causing the blood to accumulate in the channels and collaterals of the skin, which results in the skin becoming deep red and hot. Unlike a patient with psoriasis who has red, dry skin with excessive scales, this patient has dry skin with poor elasticity that is not excessively scaly. That means that at this moment, the lack of moisture in the skin (i.e., the loss of moisture from the body fluids in the skin) is more severe than its malnourishment (the loss of nourishment from the blood and yin of the body).

Diagnosis

Hot blood pattern with wind-dryness pattern caused by hot blood

The red skin and burning sensation in the skin indicate excessive heat. Itchy skin indicates that pathogenic wind has already occupied the interstices and pores, resulting in disharmony of the nutritive yin (blood) and protective yang (qi) in the skin. The dry skin and lack of elasticity indicate that the body fluids have been consumed by heat, leading to the skin losing its moisture.

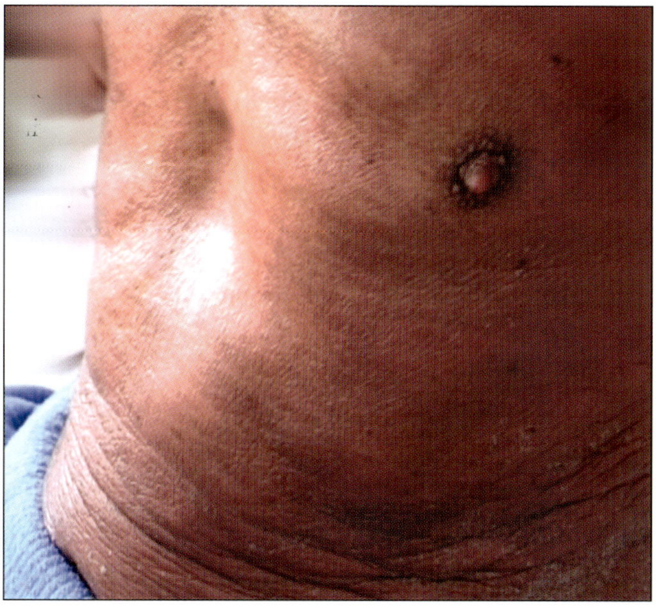

Fig. 4-9: *Drug dermatitis (allergic reaction to medication)*

The patient has deep red skin over the entire body with high skin temperature, and scales are visible on the lower back.

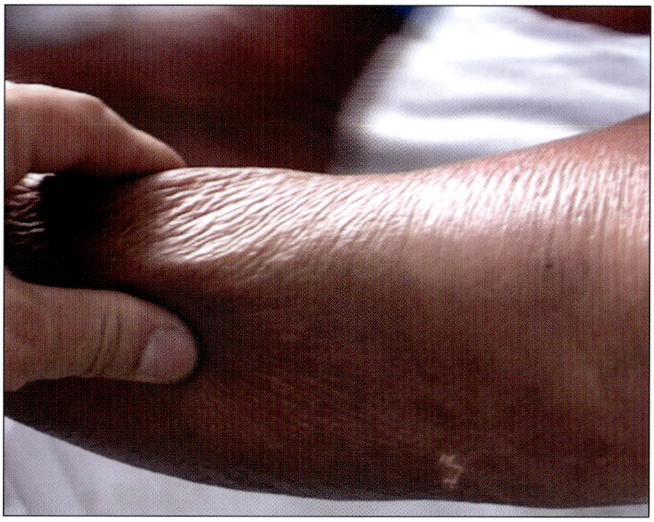

Fig. 4-10: *Same patient*

The skin on the legs is dry and lacks elasticity (poor skin turgor).

Differential diagnosis

Itchy skin can be attributed to a variety of causes. Most commonly, there is disharmony between the nutritive yin (blood) and protective yang (qi) caused by pathogenic wind. The pathogenic wind can be external or internal. The former is one of the six external pathogenic factors (or pernicious influences) and may cause hives (urticaria); the latter is internal wind created by internal dryness and is associated with xerosis. The principal point of differentiation is that external wind is accompanied by symptoms caused by exterior patterns, in which skin rashes are common, whereas internal wind is accompanied by symptoms caused by patterns of interior heat, in which skin rashes may be absent.

A medication-related allergy manifests in different types of rashes. (See the following section on rashes [Figs. 4-22 to 4-25] for more details.)

Red and Painful Skin

Clinical manifestations

Irregular patches of erythemic skin, commonly involving the lower limbs, with a burning sensation and pain. General symptoms are fever and chills. These symptoms may recur over a period of years.

Key points: See Figs. 4-11 and 4-12 (p. 57).

Pathological process

Red skin, varying from a localized skin eruption to total skin involvement, is a characteristic manifestation of patterns of hot blood. Erysipelas develops from an accumulation of pathogenic heat and manifests as local erythema in the skin. Most cases of erysipelas result from pathogenic heat toxin in the blood—caused by an invasion of external damp-heat or dampness that has accumulated over a long time that eventually transforms into heat toxin—or from pathogenic heat in the body that evolves into heat toxin.

The erythema on the skin is due to heat toxin pushing the blood to the surface of the skin. The heat toxin accumulates in the blood, causing obstruction in the local channels and collaterals such that the qi and blood cannot circulate properly; a burning sensation with severe pain and swelling thereupon develops locally. Although the skin lesion manifests within a limited area, the pathogenic heat toxin has been dispersed by the circulating blood throughout the body, causing the patient's fever and chills.

Diagnosis

Hot blood pattern, with pathogenic heat toxin in the blood

Both local and general symptoms are characterized by heat. The erythematous skin lesion indicates a pattern of hot blood. The localized skin lesion with a sharply demarcated border, burning sensation, and pain are all due to an accumulation of pathogenic heat toxins in the area. The recurring nature of the episodes indicates that the pathogenic factor is damp-heat. Because of the presence of dampness, it is a lingering, chronic, and sometimes dormant condition, which is difficult to relieve completely.

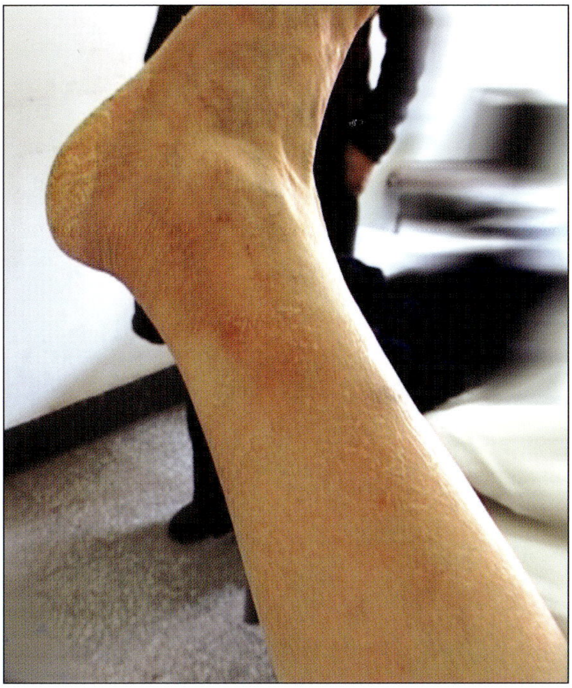

Fig. 4-11: *Erysipelas of the leg*

An erythematous and edematous skin lesion on the leg, with a sharply demarcated border between itself and normal skin

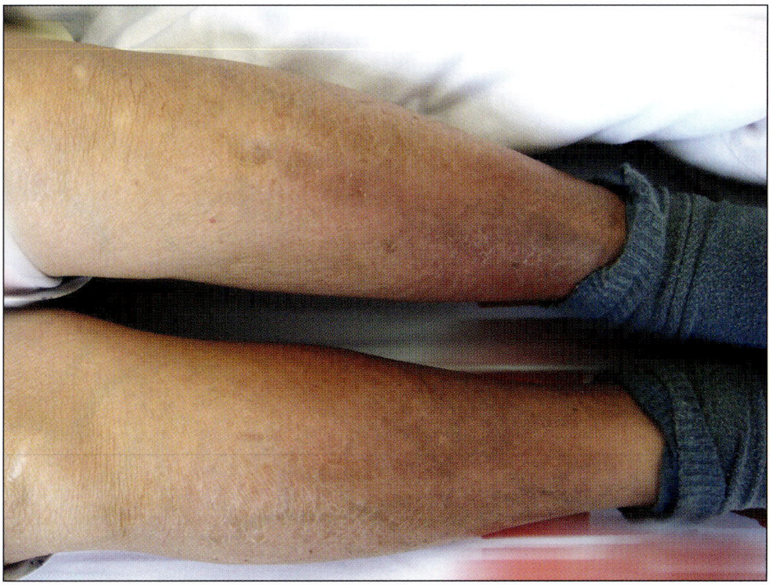

Fig. 4-12: *Chronic, recurrent erysipelas*

Erythematous and edematous skin lesions on both lower extremities. The skin is painful, swollen, and warm. The patient also experiences malaise and fever.

Differential diagnosis

A common cause of erysipelas in the lower limbs is an invasion by pathogenic dampness or damp-heat. Dampness is a yin pathogenic factor that can be due to either external invasion of pathogenic dampness or internal generation inside the body. Because pathogenic dampness resembles water, it readily sinks to the lower part of the body. Another cause is an accumulation of pathogenic heat. Some patients have a hot constitution. If dampness has the opportunity to combine with this heat, it forms damp-heat. The damp-heat develops into heat toxin, which appears as superficial dermal erythema and other symptoms.

In clinical practice, however, it is not always possible to clearly determine the initial cause of this condition. Whether due to an invasion of pathogenic damp-heat or dampness that has transformed into heat, or to an accumulation of pathogenic heat within the body, these different pathogenic factors can eventually evolve into heat toxin and present with similar symptoms. The treatment principle therefore depends on the clinical manifestations, which are mainly associated with the severity of the heat toxin. The underlying cause may be ignored.

Desquamation

Clinical manifestations

Red, dry, desquamative skin, peeling off in scales or sheets, which may be itchy.

Key points: See Figs. 4-13 through 4-16 (pp. 59-60).

Pathological process

Desquamation is a manifestation of malnourishment of the skin. This is similar to the pathological process discussed in the previous section (Figs. 4-9 and 4-10), as pathogenic heat in the blood has evaporated the body fluids and consumed the nutritive yin, resulting in the loss of moisture in the skin, which becomes dry and itchy. The pathogenic heat also disturbs the blood circulation, causing blood to accumulate in the collaterals of the skin and resulting in the skin becoming red. Desquamation and scales are the result of both malnourishment of the skin, caused by a loss of nutritive yin in the blood, as well as abnormal circulation of blood in the collaterals.

Diagnosis

Hot blood pattern, with pathogenic heat in the blood leading to dryness

Red skin indicates heat in the blood. Dryness of the skin indicates consumption of the body fluids caused by heat. Scaly and desquamative skin indicates that the skin has lost the nourishment of the yin and blood.

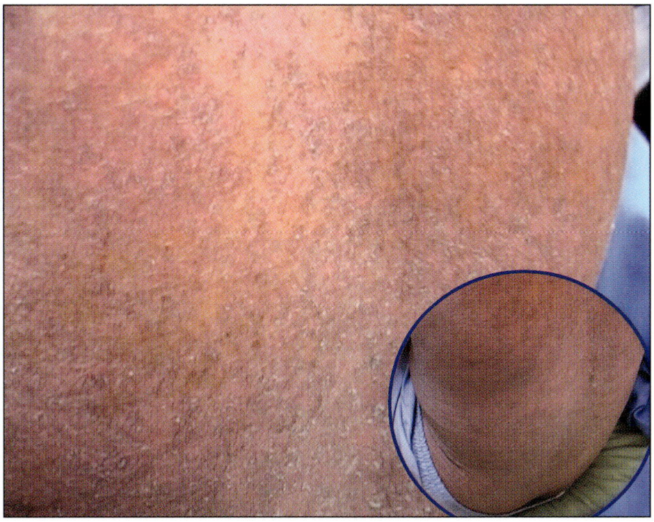

Fig. 4-13: *Psoriasis*

Red and dry skin. A large amount of small scales appear on the skin, all over the body.

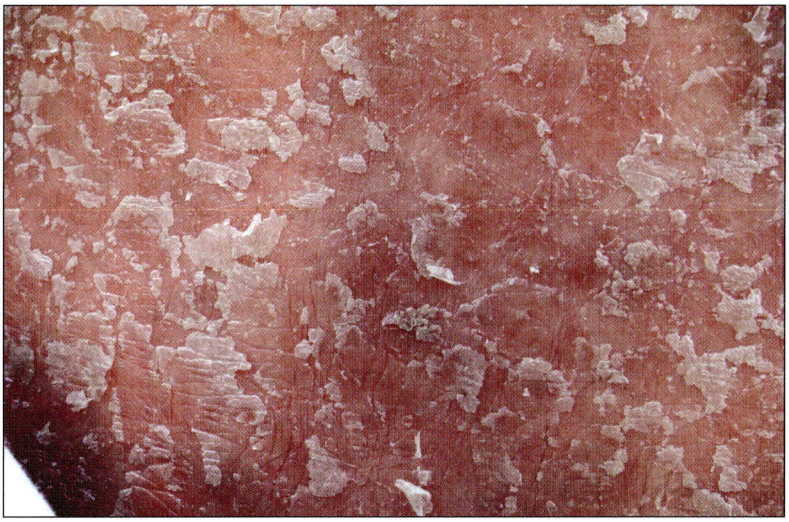

Fig. 4-14: *Severe erythroderma associated with allergic drug reactions*

The skin is diffusely erythematous with excoriations and large areas of exfoliation. The patient is shivering and the skin is hot to the touch.

Differential diagnosis

Red skin and scales are the common symptoms of skin conditions. In the first three sections of this chapter (Figs. 4-1 to 4-8), the images demonstrate changes in the color of the skin; in this section (Figs. 4-13 to 4-16), the images show desquamation.

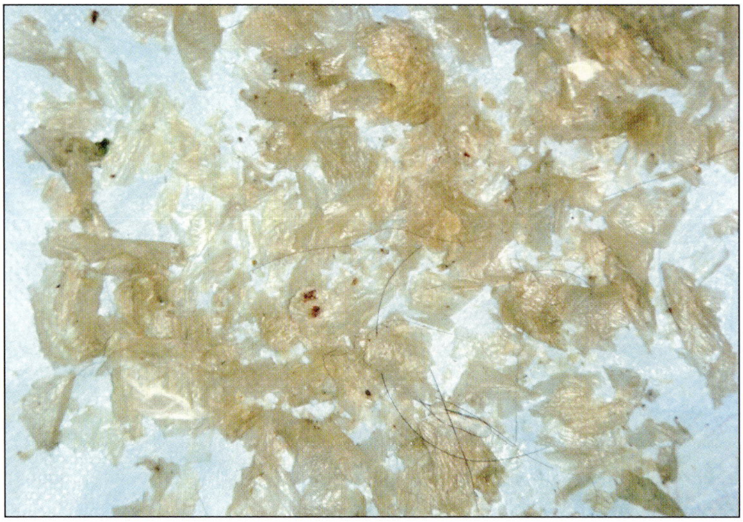

Fig. 4-15: *Same patient as above*
This photo shows flakes of detached, scaly skin.

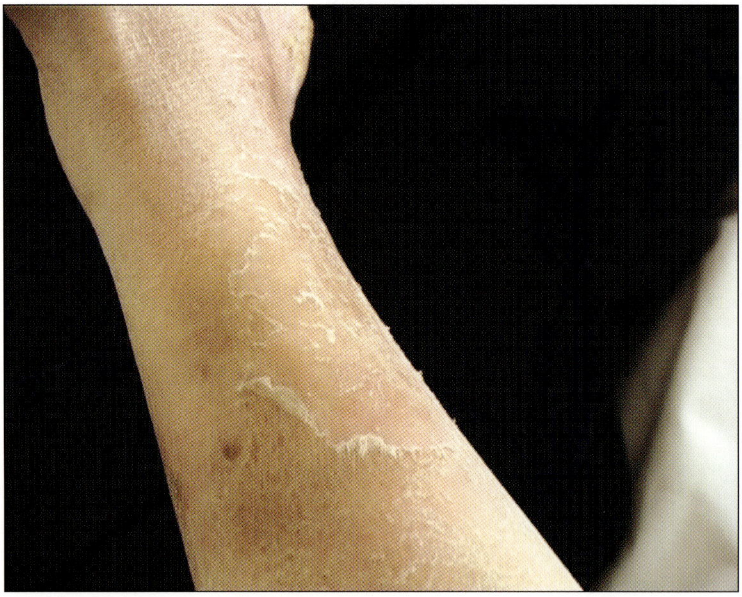

Fig. 4-16: *A patient recovering from erysipelas*
Flakes peeling off from the lower leg are visible.

In Chinese medicine these two symptoms have different pathological processes and diagnostic meanings. The change in skin color indicates a change in the flow of blood through the channels and collaterals: this reflects the severity of pathogenic heat. On the other hand, desquamation and scales are associated with malnourishment of the skin: this reflects the degree of injury to the blood and yin.

Alopecia

Clinical manifestations

Extensive and greasy dandruff on the scalp. Excessive hair loss causes a diffuse thinning of the hair.

Key points: See Figs. 4-17 and 4-18 below.

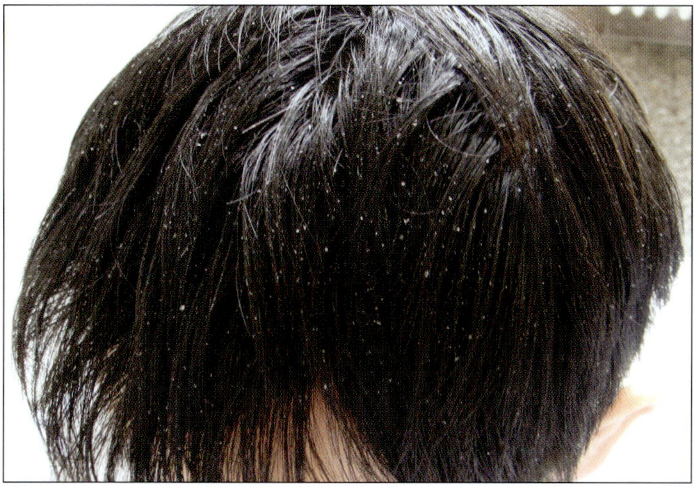

Fig. 4-17: *Seborrheic dermatitis*

Extensive and greasy dandruff on the scalp. The color of the hair is lighter than normal and has poor luster; there is obvious seborrhea.

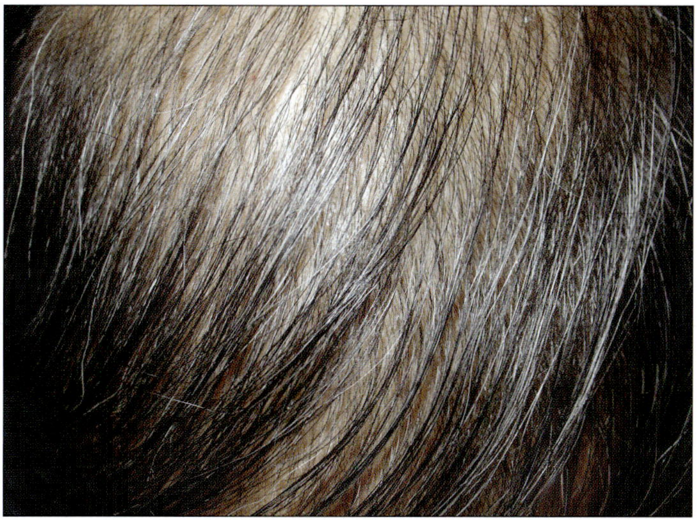

Fig. 4-18: *Another patient with seborrheic dermatitis*

This patient has general hair loss over the entire scalp. The remaining hair is thin, dry, dull, and lusterless.

Pathological process

Loss of hair is due to malnourishment in the hair from the blood. A well-known saying in Chinese medicine is that "the hair is the surplus of the blood." This means that the hair relies on nourishment from the blood to maintain its normal color, texture, and appearance.

Pathogenic heat in the blood can force the yin upward, leading to excessive secretion of sebum and a greasy feeling on the scalp. The excessive sebum can block normal qi and blood circulation in the channels and collaterals of the scalp, preventing the yang from rising; the hair thereby loses its normal luster.

This obstruction of the channels and collaterals also makes it difficult for the blood to supply sufficient moisture and nourishment to the hair, which explains why the hair becomes dry and easily falls out. The excessive shedding of dandruff is due to the malnourishment of the epidermis on the scalp.

Diagnosis

Hot blood pattern with pathogenic heat rising to disturb the scalp

The abnormal color, texture, and significant loss of hair indicate malnourishment of the hair. The dandruff indicates malnourishment of the epidermis of the scalp. The excessive sebum on the scalp reflects pathogenic heat in the blood.

Differential diagnosis

There are various causes of hair loss, most commonly blood deficiency, Kidney deficiency, or hot blood. Hair loss caused by blood deficiency has been discussed in Ch. 3; the reader is referred to that chapter for further details.

Hair loss caused by Kidney deficiency is, of course, a pattern of deficiency. This type of hair loss is often seen in middle-aged and elderly people, or in those with severe diseases. The patient has a dry rather than an oily complexion.

By contrast, hair loss due to hot blood is a pattern of excess. This condition is often encountered in young, strong people and is not associated with other diseases. The patient has an excessively copious secretion of sebum on the scalp.

Skin Infections

Clinical manifestations

Localized red, swollen, hot, suppurative, and painful skin

Key points: See Figs. 4-19 through 4-21 (pp. 63-64).

Pathological process

In Chinese medicine, *yōng yáng* (痈疡) is an inflamed area of skin that has become red, prominent, tender, and filled with pus, the same as infected skin in conventional

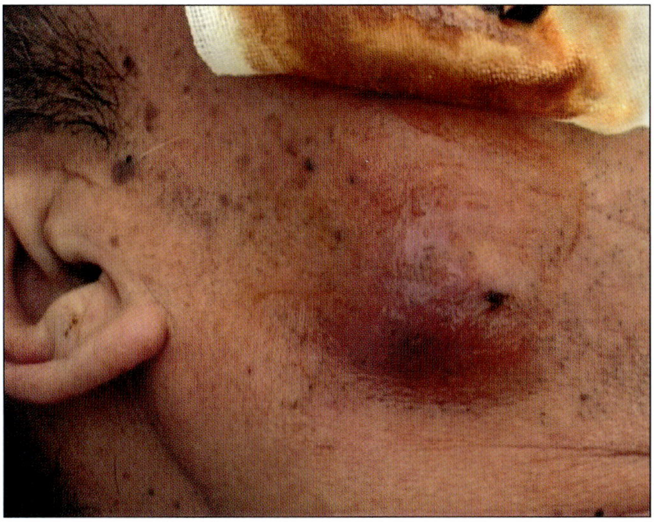

Fig. 4-19: *Furuncle on a patient's cheek*

This lesion is red, swollen, hot and tender, and topped by a pyogenic head.

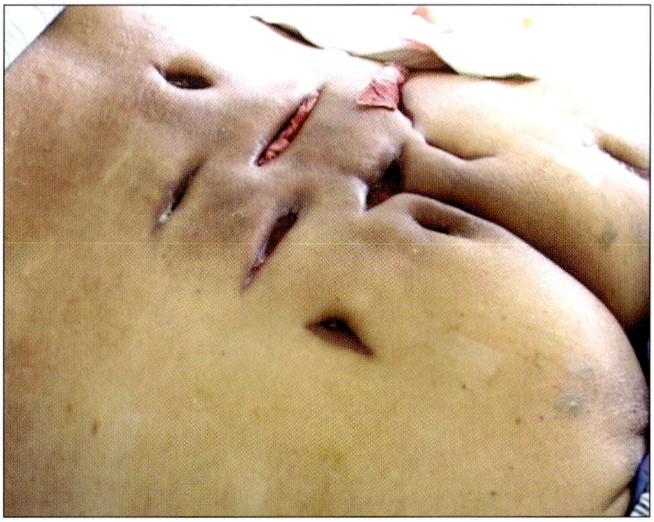

Fig. 4-20: *Diabetic patient with a carbuncle on the lower back*

The abscess has been lanced and the pus drained. The photo is a close-up of the abscess after surgical incisions were made.

medicine. But the explanation of the causes and pathological processes is very different. In Chinese medical theory, the main causes of infected skin are pathogenic damp-heat, fire toxin, and hot blood.

Damp-heat, derived either from the environment or from internal disorders, is a heavy and viscous pathogenic factor that impedes the circulation of qi. It causes

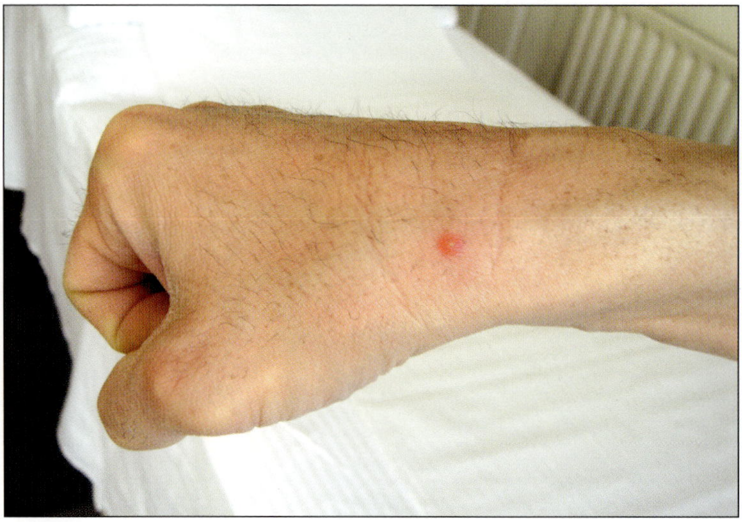

Fig. 4-21: *A case of recurrent folliculitis*

A single follicular pustule, topped by a suppurating head, can be seen on the patient's wrist.

stagnation in the body; heat develops from this stagnation and is then transformed into fire toxin.

Pathogenic heat, which also originates from either inside or outside the body, can reach the blood level and cause hot blood patterns. The heat forces the blood so that it is concentrated in the inflamed skin, which then becomes red, swollen, and puffy. Fire toxin rots the accumulated blood and dead tissue in the inflamed area and turns them into pus.

Diagnosis

Hot blood pattern with accumulated, clumped fire toxin and damp-heat

In Chinese medicine and ancient philosophy, extreme heat transforms into fire. Fire toxin is a highly-concentrated pathogenic heat factor. The process of suppuration is associated with retention of damp-heat and fire toxin. Localized swelling, heat, and redness in the skin indicate that a strong fire toxin has developed in the skin. Pain and tenderness indicate an obstruction of the channels and collaterals caused by stagnation of qi and blood.

Suppuration indicates accumulated, clumped damp-heat and fire toxin. A larger abscess with red, prominent, hot, tender, and painful skin, together with excessive pus, indicate a severe accumulation of damp-heat and fire toxin that is called a toxic swelling (*zhǒng dú* 肿毒) in Chinese medicine.

Differential diagnosis

Interestingly, in both Chinese and Western medicine, the same terms are used for skin infections. However, there are some differences in conception. In Western medicine, folliculitis refers to a superficially infected follicle, while a furuncle is regarded as a more deep-set, follicle-based infection. A carbuncle is made of several joined furuncles.

In Chinese medicine, folliculitis does not exist as a name for a disease; folliculitis and furuncles both pertain to *jiē* 疖 (furuncle or boil), while *yōng* (痈) is similar to a carbuncle in Western medicine. As *jiē* (furuncle) and *yōng* (carbuncle) have the same causes and pathological processes, the names refer only to the different stages of the disease.

Rashes

Clinical manifestations

General skin rashes with dense, tiny, bright red papules on the skin. The rashes are slightly elevated. Itchy and hot sensations are common.

Key points: See Figs. 4-22 through 4-25 (pp. 66-67).

Pathological process

Skin rashes are symptomatic of an overflow of the collaterals (blood vessels). The heat accelerates the circulation of blood and significantly increases the amount of blood in the channels and collaterals. The huge cutaneous blood flow causes bright red skin over a large area of the body.

This bright color changes when pressure is applied to the skin: it disappears under pressure and returns when the pressure is released. This phenomenon is evidence of congestion rather than subcutaneous bleeding, which in Chinese medicine suggests pathogenic heat in the nutritive level (nutritive level pattern) rather than in the blood level (blood level pattern).

Pathogenic heat and blood collect in the interstices and pores, which become prominent and develop into dense papules on the surface (skin rashes). The pathogenic heat that has accumulated in the interstices and pores is spread outward through the skin, as evidenced by the rash, partially relieving the damage to the skin caused by the pathogenic heat. Therefore, apart from the papules, the skin turgor or flexibility is normal, and there is no evidence of scales or dryness.

Diagnosis

Hot blood pattern with accumulation of pathogenic heat in the nutritive level

Bright red papules indicate a hot blood pattern. Prominent papules indicate a collection of pathogenic heat in the interstices and pores of the skin, affecting the superficial collaterals. Because pressure causes the color to disappear, this indicates that the collaterals are not damaged and that the blood can continue to flow within them.

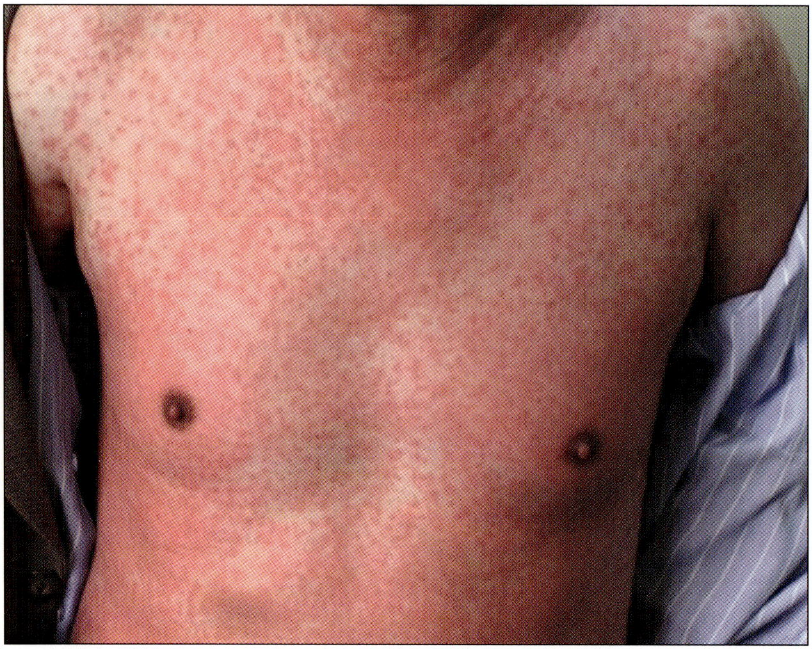

Fig. 4-22: *Drug eruption*

Numerous tiny papules are spread over the upper back and chest.

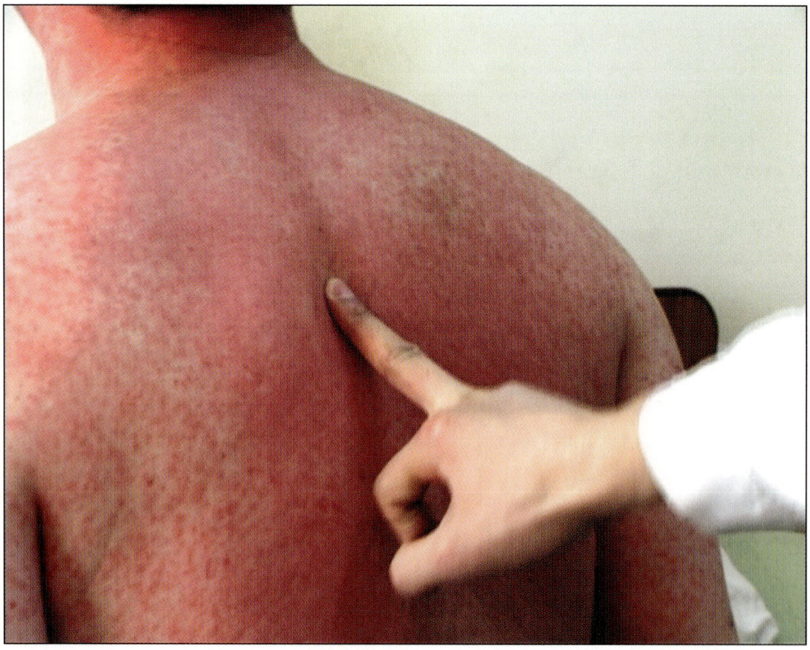

Fig. 4-23: *Same patient's back*

Digital pressure is applied to the skin.

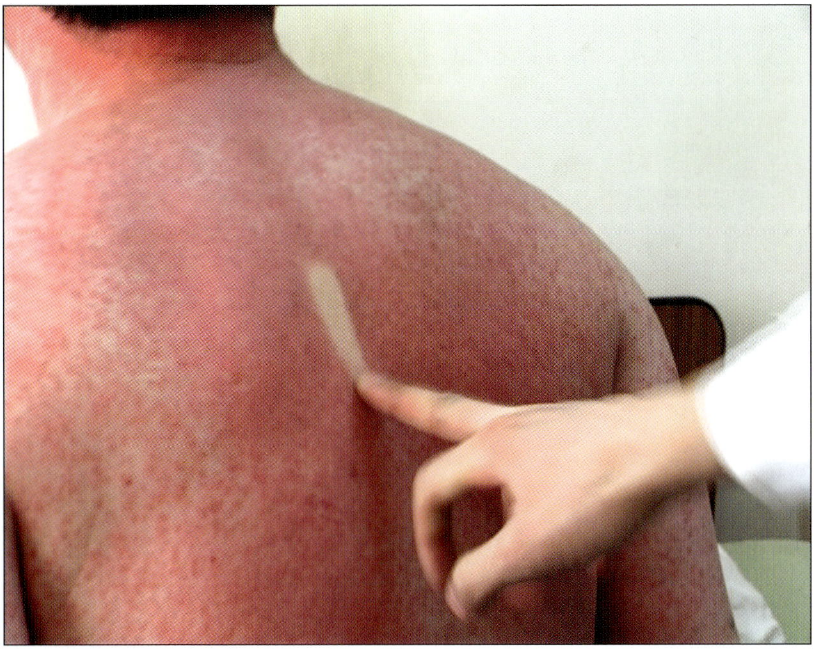

Fig. 4-24: *Same patient*

Disappearance of the redness is visible immediately after pressure is released.

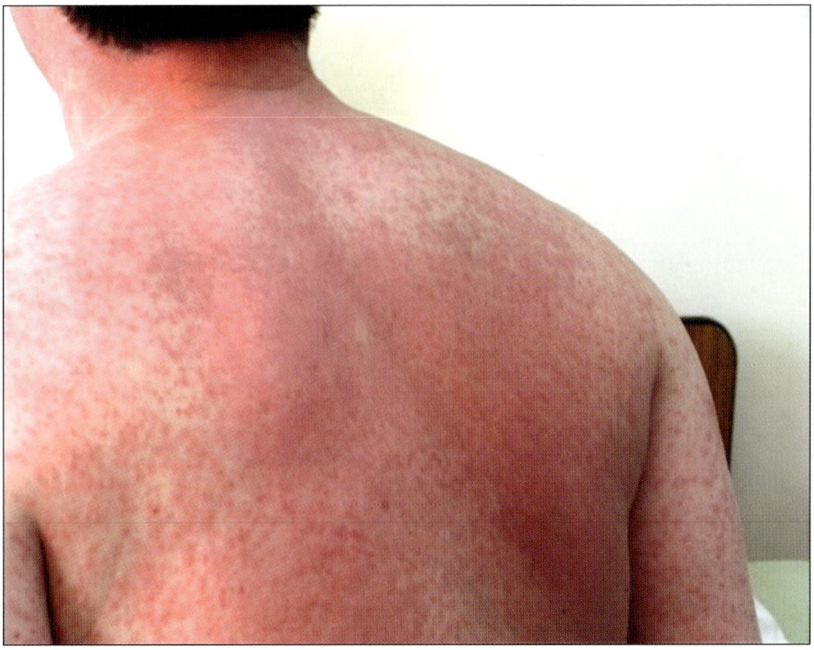

Fig. 4-25: *Same patient*

The patient's skin reveals recovery of the color from pressure and return of the redness.

Differential diagnosis

As noted earlier, in Chinese medicine there are two stages of hot blood patterns that are distinguished by the depth of the heat invasion: pathogenic heat reaches the nutritive level or the blood level. The former is relatively mild, and the latter is more severe. Diagnosis of these two levels must take into account the manifestations on the skin, the general signs and symptoms, and the tongue and pulse. Skin rashes are common and are of significance for differentiation.

Rashes associated with nutritive level patterns have raised lesions and are called *zhěn* (疹) in Chinese medicine. They more or less resemble papules in conventional medicine. They are characterized by a small, conical, and clustered elevation of the skin that can be felt when the skin is touched. Pressure applied to the skin results in the disappearance of the red coloration, as in this case.

Rashes associated with blood level patterns are flat lesions named *bān* (斑) in Chinese medicine, which describes a rash that is similar to macules in conventional medicine. Macules or *bān* are scattered, grouped, or confluent lesions; they consist of a small or large discolored area of the skin and they are flat. They can only be seen and not felt. Pressure applied on the skin does not change its color. Examples of these can be seen in this chapter in the photos of patients with hemorrhage (Figs. 4-26 and 4-27), and also in Figs. 6-12 and 6-13 of Ch. 6 on blood stasis, as well as in Fig. 2-19 of Ch. 2 on qi deficiency.

Drug-induced eruptions can manifest in a variety of skin conditions such as rash, erythema, maculopapular rash, blisters, pustules, hives, and erythroderma. According to traditional Chinese medical differentiation, some of these conditions belong to patterns of heat in the nutritive level, some to patterns of heat in the blood level, and some to patterns which may be different from hot blood patterns, such as chicken pox, which is often associated with pathogenic dampness or damp-heat. Thus the drug eruption should be diagnosed in Chinese medicine based on the appearance of its skin rash and the general symptoms.

Hemorrhage

Clinical manifestations

Medical bleeding (bleeding not associated with trauma). Bleeding, which can be caused by different medical conditions, can occur internally or externally.

Key points: See Figs. 4-26 through 4-28 (pp. 69-70).

Scarlet Tongue

A red or deep red tongue is associated with hot blood patterns. (For more information, see Ch. 8 on tongue diagnosis.)

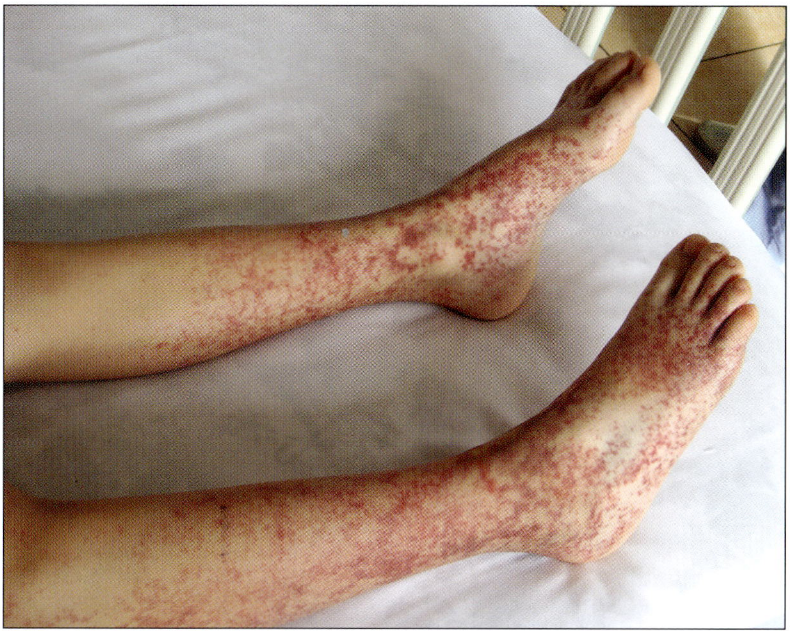

Fig. 4-26: *Henoch-Schönlein purpura (HSP), or allergic purpura*

Red or purple bruises have developed on the legs. The young patient complains of abdominal pain accompanied by blood in the stools.

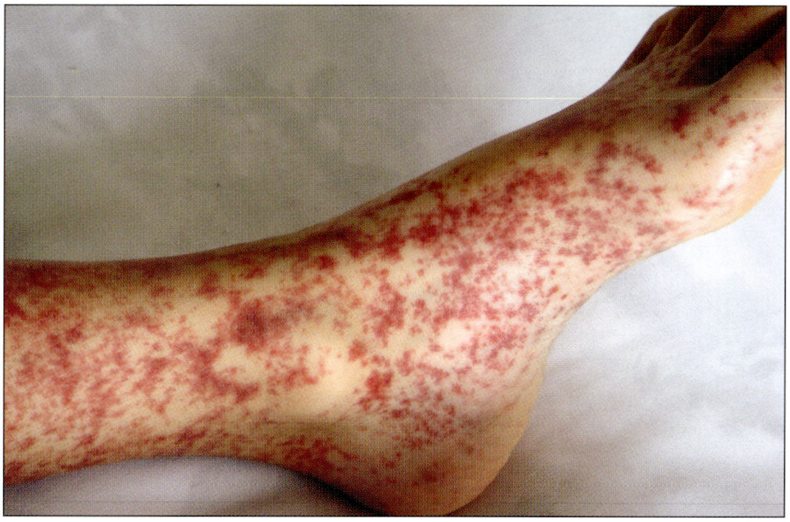

Fig. 4-27: *Same patient*

A close view of the bruises. These are dense, deep red bruises that do not disappear when pressure is applied to the skin.

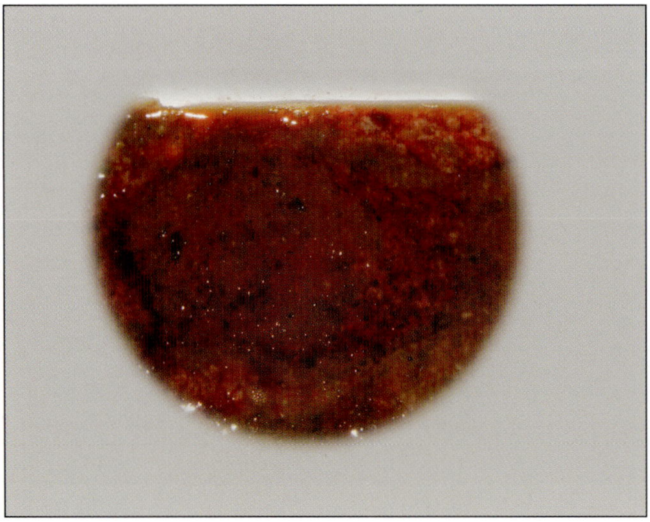

Fig. 4-28: *Ulcerative colitis*

The patient has abdominal pain and diarrhea. The image displays feces mixed with blood and mucus. (See Ch. 7 on bleeding patterns for further details.)

Summary

Table 4-1: *Key diagnostic points for patterns of hot blood*

Cause of Symptoms	Symptoms (Images)	Examples of Diseases and Symptoms
Excessive accumulation of blood in the collaterals on the surface of the body	Bright red skin, dense papules or erythema (Figs. 4-1 to 4-12, and 4-22 to 4-25)	Infectious diseases (e.g., septicemia), hematologic diseases (e.g., leukemia), skin conditions (e.g., psoriasis, drug eruption, erysipelas, erythroderma)
Pathogenic heat disturbance of Heart and mind	High fever, anxiety, insomnia, unconsciousness	Infectious diseases of the neurological system (e.g., meningitis, viral encephalitis), mental disorders (e.g., anxiety, psychoses); other: premenstrual syndrome, menopausal disorders

—continued next page

Cause of Symptoms	Symptoms (Images)	Examples of Diseases and Symptoms
Pathogenic heat blocking and rotting the qi, blood, and tissues	Pyogenic infections with suppuration; red, hot, raised, painful skin (Figs. 4-19 to 4-21)	Bacterial infections, skin and soft tissue infection (e.g., furuncle, carbuncle, abscess, infected wound), purulence in internal organs (e.g., pleural empyema, intra-abdominal abscesses); other factors (e.g., diabetes-related infections)
Chaotic movement of hot blood	Hemorrhage: bright red blood originating internally or externally (Figs. 4-26 to 4-28)	Hemoptysis (e.g., pulmonary TB), hematemesis (e.g. bleeding ulcer), hematologic diseases (e.g., leukemia), menorrhagia (e.g., dysfunctional uterine bleeding); other hemorrhaging (e.g., epistaxis, gingival hemorrhage, brain hemorrhage, retinal hemorrhage, hematuria)
Excessive heat leading to stirring of internal wind	High fever, unconsciousness, and convulsions	Febrile convulsions, CNS infections (e.g., meningitis)
Patterns of internal dryness caused by hot blood	Dry, thickened, and cracked skin with desquamation (flaky skin) (Figs. 4-1 to 4-6, and 4-13 to 4-16)	Skin conditions (e.g., psoriasis, recovery stage of erysipelas, or scarlet fever)
Internal wind generated from dry patterns caused by hot blood	Dry and itchy skin (Figs. 4-9 and 4-10)	Skin conditions (e.g., xerosis, psoriasis, eczema, senile pruritus)
Heat surges upward, causing blockage in the scalp and malnourishment of the hair	Excessive dandruff, excessive hair loss, and thinning of the hair (Figs. 4-17 and 4-18)	Seborrheic dermatitis
Tongue and pulse	Scarlet tongue, rapid or thin, wiry, and rapid pulse (Figs. 8-5 and 8-6)	

Acupuncture point selection principles:

Clear the heat and cool the blood

Selection of points:

GV-14, LI-4, SP-10, GB-34, BL-40

Manipulation method:

Reducing and bleeding method

Point selection for complications:

- To clear heat from the Heart: PC-3
- To calm the spirit and open the orifices: GV-26, PC-6, M-UE-1 (use bleeding method)
- To clear heat and extinguish wind: GV-26, GV-16, SI-3, BL-40
- To stop bleeding: PC-4, LU-6
- To enrich the yin and moisten dryness: SP-10, SP-6, BL-17

Table 4-2: *Acupuncture treatment*

Points	Point Explanation	Point Combinations
GV-14	The meeting point of the seven yang channels, this is very effective for removing pathogenic heat.	The combination of GV-14 and LI-4 forms a strong pair for removing both exterior and/or interior heat.
LI-4	Good for clearing heat, expelling wind, and relieving exterior patterns.	
SP-10	The Chinese name for SP-10 is "sea of blood." It removes the heat from the blood in the entire body.	
GB-34	The sea point of the leg lesser yang Gallbladder channel, this is also the influential point for the sinews. It clears heat and regulates the sinews.	This pair is chosen to relax the sinews, remove obstructions from the channel, and check internal wind.
BL-40	Cools the blood and releases heat.	

Treatment principle:

Clear heat from the nutritive level or cool the blood

Table 4-3: *Treatment with herbal formulas*

HERB AND DOSAGE	FLAVORS AND NATURE	ASSOCIATED CHANNELS	FORMULA ANALYSIS

■ **Rhinoceros Horn and Rehmannia Decoction** *(xī jiăo dì huáng tāng)*

COOLS THE BLOOD

HERB AND DOSAGE	FLAVORS AND NATURE	ASSOCIATED CHANNELS	FORMULA ANALYSIS
Bubali Cornu *(shuĭ niú jiăo)*, 30g	Bitter, salty, and cold	Heart and Liver	Clears heat from the nutritive level and cools the blood
Rehmanniae Radix *(shēng dì huáng)*, 30g	Sweet, bitter, and cold	Heart, Liver, and Kidney	Clears heat, cools the blood, and nourishes the yin
Moutan Cortex *(mŭ dān pí)*, 9g	Bitter, acrid, and cold	Heart, Liver, and Kidney	Both herbs cool the blood, regulate the circulation of blood, and remove blood stasis.
Paeoniae Radix rubra *(chì sháo)*, 12g	Bitter and slightly cold	Liver	

■ **Clear the Nutritive Level Decoction** *(qīng yíng tāng)*

CLEARS HEAT FROM THE NUTRITIVE LEVEL

HERB AND DOSAGE	FLAVORS AND NATURE	ASSOCIATED CHANNELS	FORMULA ANALYSIS
Bubali Cornu *(shuĭ niú jiăo)*	Bitter, salty, and cold	Heart and Liver	Both substances clear heat from the nutritive level and cool the blood.
Rehmanniae Radix *(shēng dì huáng)*, 15g	Sweet, bitter, and cold	Heart, Liver, and Kidney	
Scrophulariae Radix *(xuán shēn)*, 9g	Bitter, salty, and cold	Lung, Stomach, and Kidney	These two herbs plus two above clear heat and nourish the yin.
Ophiopogonis Radix *(mài mén dōng)*, 9g	Sweet and cold	Lung, Heart, and Stomach	

—*continued next page*

HERB AND DOSAGE	FLAVORS AND NATURE	ASSOCIATED CHANNELS	FORMULA ANALYSIS
Salviae miltiorrhizae Radix *(dān shēn)*, 6g	Bitter and cold	Heart and Liver	Cools the blood and dispels blood stasis
Coptidis Rhizoma *(huáng lián)*, 4.5g	Bitter and cold	Heart, Liver, and Stomach	Clears heat from the qi level and drains fire
Lophatheri Herba *(dàn zhú yè)*, 3g	Sweet, bland, and cold	Heart, Lung, and Stomach	Move heat from the nutritive level to the qi level and then out of the skin
Lonicerae Flos *(jīn yín huā)*, 9g	Sweet and cold	Lung and Stomach	
Forsythiae Fructus *(lián qiáo)*, 6g	Bitter and cold	Lung and Heart	

CHAPTER 5

Patterns of Cold Blood

Cold and Blue-Purple (Cyanosis) or White Skin

Clinical manifestations

A bluish discoloration of the skin that worsens when the temperature is cold. Another manifestation is that the skin on the hands or feet first turns white, then blue or purple, and this is accompanied by a cold, numb, or painful sensation in the affected extremities. The color change is usually a response to cold.

Key points: See Figs. 5-1 through 5-3 (pp. 75-76).

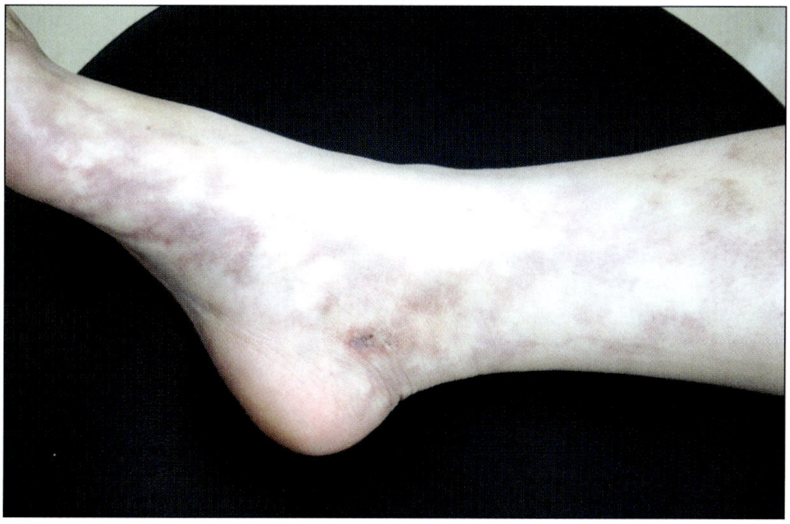

Fig. 5-1: *Livedoid vasculitis (livedo reticularis)*

A blue lace-like area of the skin in the lower extremities. The condition can be aggravated by exposure to cold.

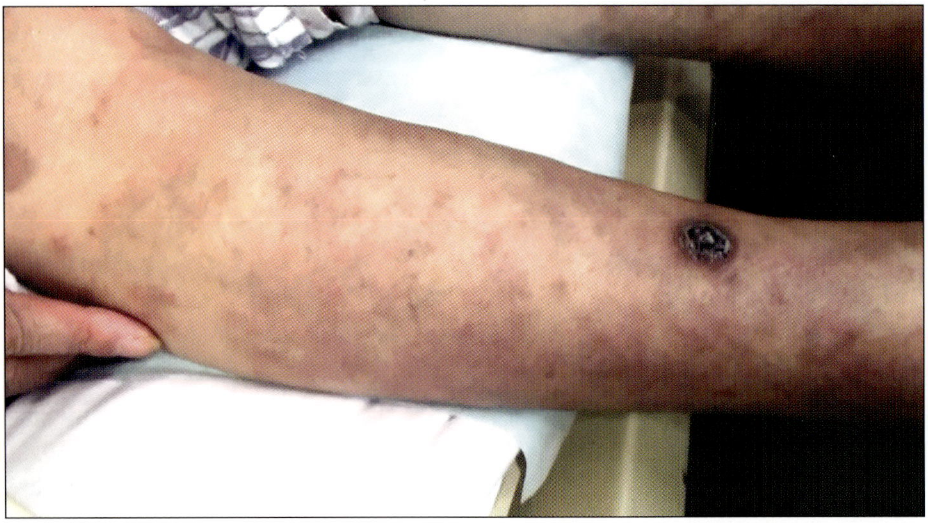

Fig. 5-2: *Another case of livedoid vasculitis*

A purple lace-like area of the skin with painful ulceration occurring in the lower leg

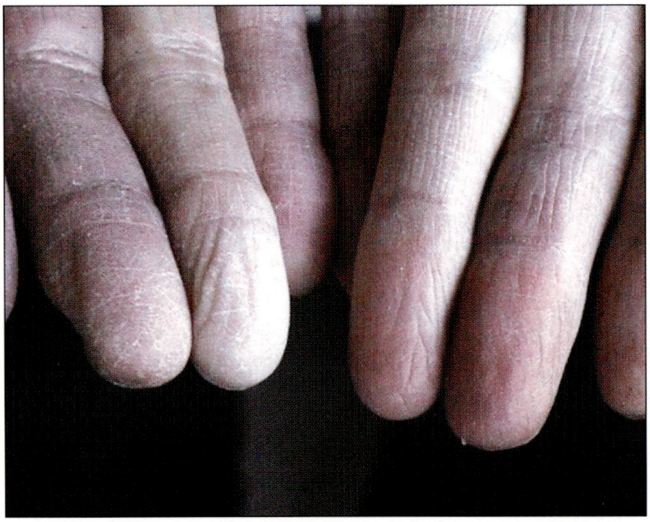

Fig. 5-3: *Raynaud's syndrome*

One finger on the patient's right hand has turned white soon after both hands were exposed to cold.

Pathological process

Blue or purple skin indicates poor circulation of blood in the collaterals.

It is well known that pathogenic cold is one of the yin pathogenic factors that damages the yang qi of the body. When the extremities have a very small supply of yang qi, the hands and feet become cold. Pathogenic cold congeals or "freezes" the blood such that the blood becomes clotted within the collaterals, resulting in blood stasis, and hence the fingers first turn white, then blue-purple. Pathogenic cold constricts the vessels and slows down the circulation of qi and blood, leading to an obstruction in the collaterals and then pain.

Diagnosis

A pattern of cold blood with pathogenic cold congeals the blood in the collaterals

The cold and painful extremities triggered by a cold environment indicate an invasion of pathogenic cold. The cold and white skin indicates poor circulation in the affected area. The blue-purple skin indicates blood stasis in the collaterals. The invasion of pathogenic cold into the body affects the circulation of the qi and blood, which clearly indicates a pattern of cold blood.

Differential diagnosis

The characteristic change in color of the skin is evidence of livedo reticularis or Raynaud's syndrome in conventional medicine, but in Chinese medicine it can indicate either blood stasis or cold blood. A sensation of coldness with an associated color change is the basic evidence needed to support a diagnosis of pathogenic cold congealing the blood in patterns of cold blood in Chinese medicine. This would include livedoid vasculitis or livedo reticularis, Raynaud's syndrome, chilblains, or poor circulation.

Cold and Black Skin

Clinical manifestations

Changes in skin color and skin temperature. The skin color can be purple, bronze, or black, and is accompanied by a cold sensation. In severe cases, patients may develop a loss of sensitivity, skin ulceration, or a complication of necrosis in the affected extremity.

Key points: See Figs. 5-4 and 5-5 (p. 78).

Pathological process

Black skin indicates an obstruction to the circulation of blood.

Pathogenic cold can be external or internal. External pathogenic cold refers to cold from the environment invading the body, as in the case discussed above. Internal pathogenic cold is a pattern of yang deficiency generated by an internal disorder. Both external and internal cold have similar symptoms but patients with yang deficiency (interior cold) have symptoms that are less related to changes in the weather. The patient discussed in this section has a pattern of interior cold.

In Chinese medicine the limbs are regarded as the extremities of the yang. This implies that the yang qi in the distal part of the limbs is weaker than that within the trunk and hence more easily affected by a disorder of the yang qi. When cold is

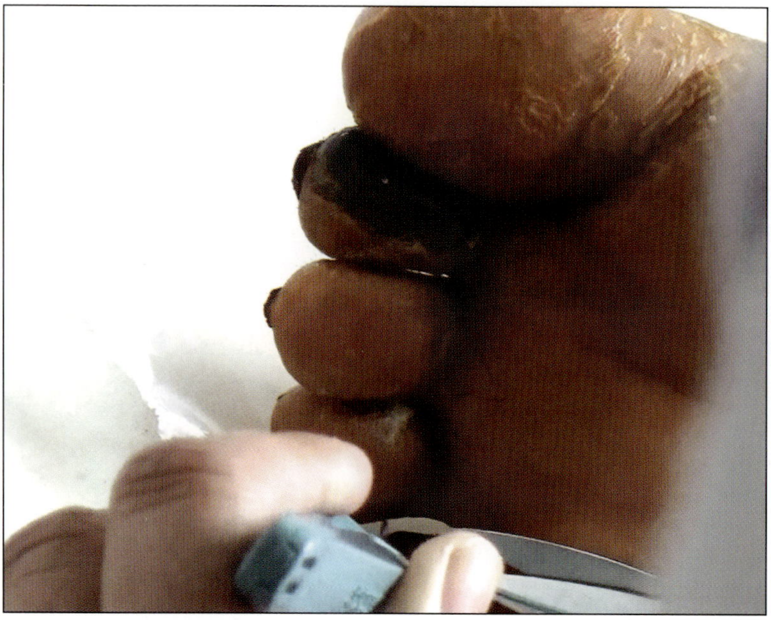

Fig. 5-4: *Diabetic foot ulcer*

The skin of the toe is purple (or bronze) in color with a black tip.

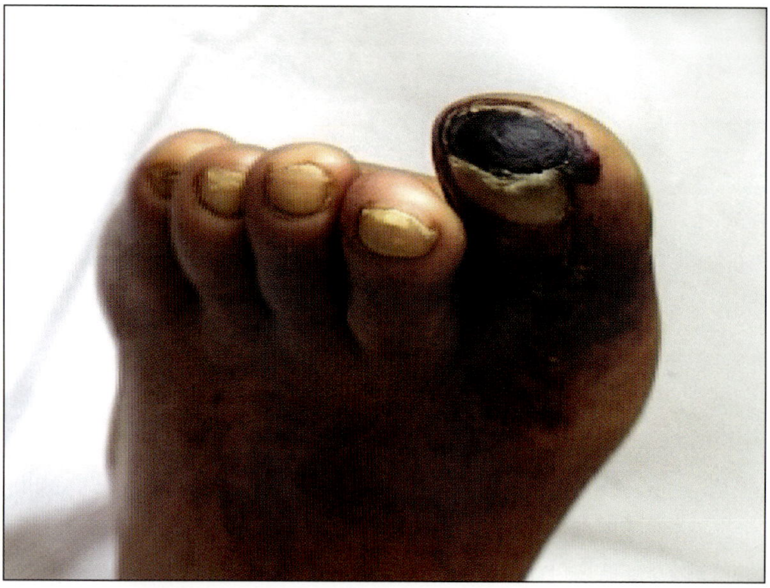

Fig. 5-5: *Another case of diabetic foot ulcer*

This image shows an ulcer covered by a black scab on the tip of the toe.

generated from yang deficiency, the symptoms begin at the weakest point of the yang qi, in this case the toes. The weakened yang qi cannot warm the extremities, which is why the feet become cold. Cold congeals the blood, causing blood stasis that blocks the circulation of blood in the channels, resulting in dark coloration of the skin and pain. Progressive impairment of the blood and yang qi supply severely compromises the function of the skin, resulting in skin ulceration.

Diagnosis

A pattern of cold blood with pathogenic cold congealing the blood in the channels

The purple (or bronze) coloration of the toes indicates blood stasis. The cold and pain in the toes indicate that the cause of the blood stasis here is pathogenic cold. This is therefore a pattern of cold blood. The ulcer and black scab on the toes indicate prolonged blood stasis and obstruction in the channels and collaterals, which is quite severe.

Differential diagnosis

Although the cold in this case is internal cold, which is different from the previous case, the pathological processes are similar in both cases. Here, pathogenic cold is constantly constricting the channels without relief and thus the prolonged blood stasis has almost blocked the channels and collaterals in the toes. The coloration of the skin in this case is therefore darker than in the previous case, demonstrating that the condition here is worse.

Gangrene

Clinical manifestations

Cold sensation and pain in the limbs. Loss of sensitivity, death of tissue (necrosis), skin ulceration, blackness, and ultimately gangrene in the affected extremity. In the worst case, this can result in amputation of the damaged extremities.

Key points: See Figs. 5-6 through 5-9 (pp. 80-81).

Pathological process

Gangrene indicates a total obstruction of the blood circulation in the channels.

Yang qi and blood (yin) play different roles in the body. The blood provides the nutrition while the yang qi supplies warmth and energy to circulate the blood to the entire body, including the organs and tissues. Pathogenic cold injures the yang qi of the extremities, causing the feet to lose warmth and become cold. Pathogenic cold slows down the circulation and congeals the blood, leading to a formation of blood stasis and an obstruction in the channels and collaterals. Blood stasis manifests in purple, bronze, or black skin coloration and the obstruction generates pain. Severe obstruction of the channels leads to a complete blockage of the blood circulation, which means a permanently arrested blood flow to the affected area, and finally a sloughing off of the gangrenous tissue.

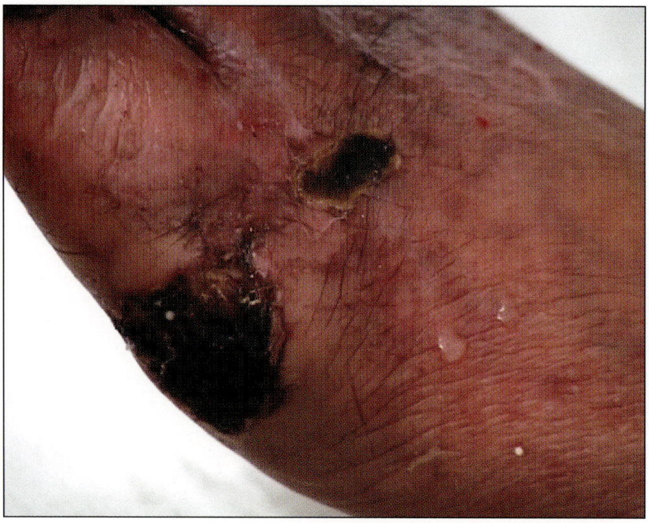

Fig. 5-6: *Thromboangiitis obliterans (Buerger's disease)*
Purple (or bronze) skin on the foot; black skin ulcers

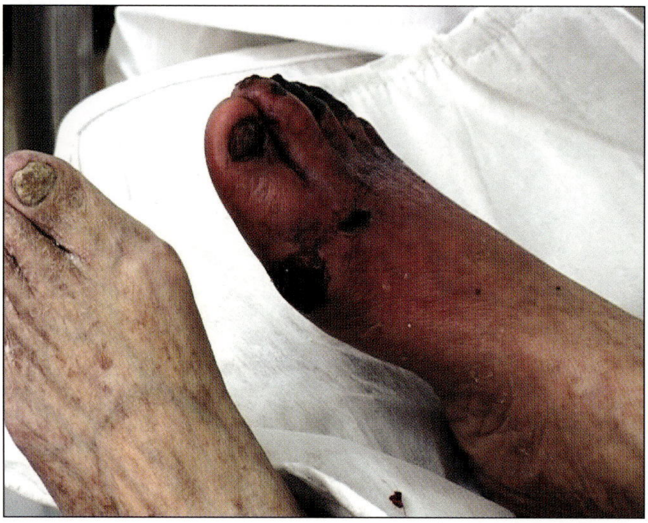

Fig. 5-7: *Same patient as above*
The image shows a comparison between the two feet.

Diagnosis

A pattern of cold blood with obstruction of the channels

Black skin indicates severe blood stasis in the channels and collaterals. The cold and pain in the foot, and the loss of sensitivity, indicate that the blood stasis is caused by pathogenic cold. The skin ulceration, necrosis, and gangrene reflect a total obstruction of qi and blood in the channels and collaterals, which is a severe stage in the pattern of cold blood.

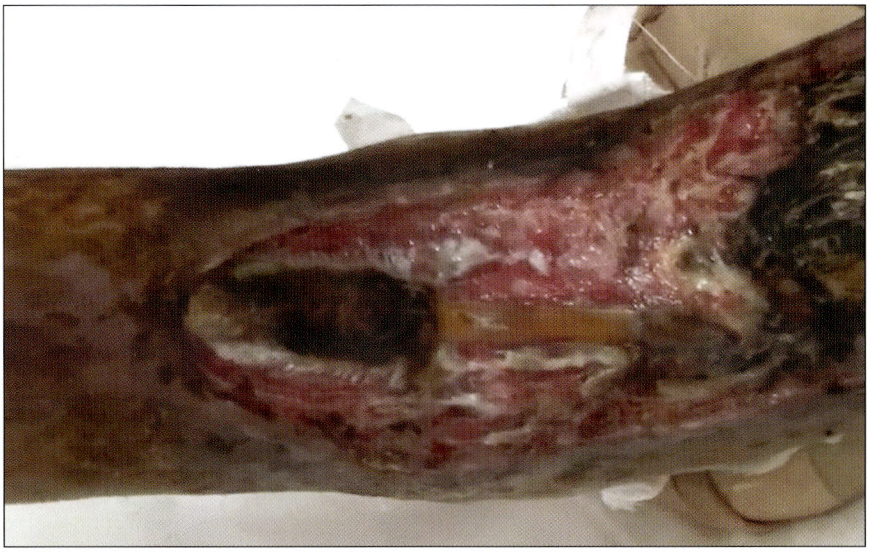

Fig. 5-8: *Atherosclerotic peripheral arterial disease*
Ulcers and necrosis in the foot. The color of the affected foot is dark black and resembles mummified flesh.

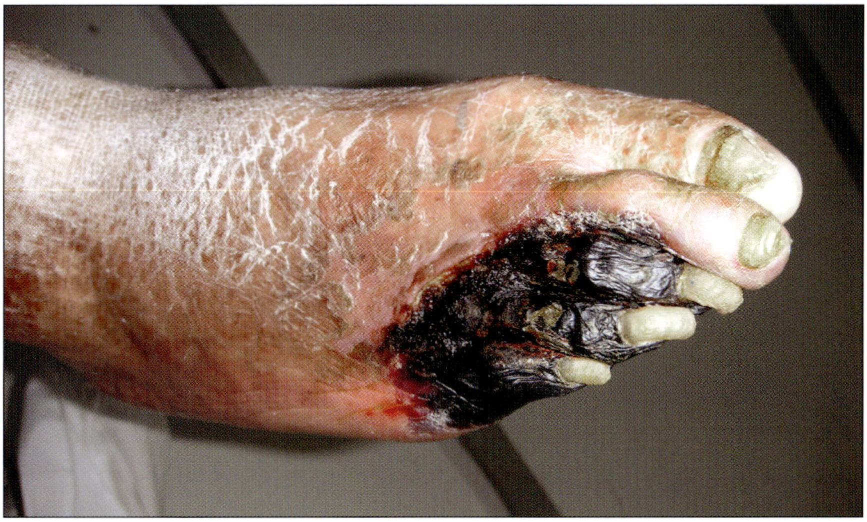

Fig. 5-9: *Diabetic ulceration with gangrene*
The patient has black toes.

Differential diagnosis

The three groups of images (Figs. 5-1 to 5-9) show the different stages of cold blood patterns, ranging from temporary and reversible to severe and permanent, and demonstrate how pathogenic cold damages the circulation of blood in the body.

According to conventional medicine, a skin ulcer of the lower extremities can be arterial or venous. In Chinese medicine, skin ulcers (also gangrene) caused by cold blood are dry and therefore categorized as arterial ulcers. Other ulcers, such as venous ulcers like stasis dermatitis or infections, in which there is secretion or suppuration on the surface, are characteristic of dampness or damp-heat rather than cold.

Tender and Deformed Joints

Clinical manifestations

Joints become swollen, tender, and stiff. This is most commonly encountered in small joints like those of the hands and feet. The pain can be relieved by warmth and is aggravated by cold. Deformed joints are common.

Key points: See Fig. 5-10 below.

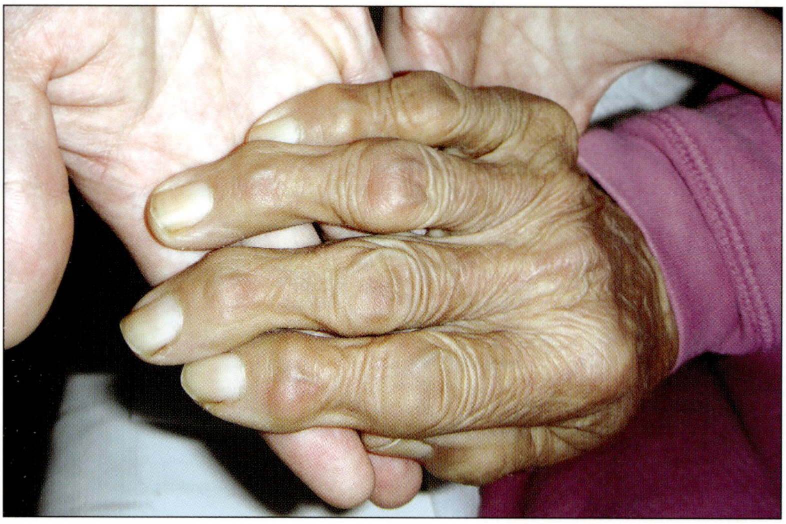

Fig. 5-10: *Rheumatoid arthritis*

This shows obvious deformation of the small joints of the hands, which have restricted movement.

Pathological process

Tenderness and deformity in the joints are evidence of an obstruction in the channels and collaterals. Qi and blood circulate in the body through the channel system. Invasion of pathogenic factors from the enviroment causes obstruction in the channels and collaterals and stagnation of qi and blood. Pathogenic cold and/or dampness are the most common factors in the clinic.

Pathogenic cold is characterized by constriction and stagnation. It blocks the circulation of qi as well as the warming of yang in the channels, causing pain and cold. The small joints located at the distal parts of the limbs, with the weakest supply of yang qi, are the most vulnerable and thus the symptoms emerge first in the fingers. Cold makes the stagnation worse and warmth improves the circulation. This explains why painful fingers worsen with cold but ease in warm surroundings. Pathogenic cold also congeals the blood in the channels, causing stiffness and swelling as malnourishment occurs in the affected areas. As time goes by, the condition worsens, leading finally to deformity and restricted movement of the joints and fingers.

Diagnosis

A pattern of cold blood with pathogenic cold constricting the channels and collaterals

The painful fingers indicate an obstruction in the channels and collaterals. The cold and painful extremities triggered by a cold environment reflect an invasion by pathogenic cold. The stiff and deformed joints indicate the presence of blood stasis in the channels and collaterals and malnourishment of the joints. The invasion of pathogenic cold into the channels and collaterals causing blood stasis indicates a pattern of cold blood.

Differential diagnosis

Arthritis (*bì* 痹 syndrome in Chinese medicine) is very commonly seen in the clinic, both in conventional and Chinese medicine. There are different types of arthritis (or *bì* syndrome) and each has a different cause. It is clinically evident that in those patients who suffer from painful joints, pathogenic cold plays an important role. Other causes include an invasion of dampness or wind, or deficiency of blood or yin, or both.

Generally speaking, in its early stage, rheumatoid arthritis is caused by an invasion of cold or dampness, or both. Degenerative joint disease and advanced stages of rheumatoid arthritis are associated with deficiency as well as with an invasion by pathogenic environmental factors. Migratory polyarthritis, one of the major criteria for supporting the diagnosis of rheumatic fever, is thought to be caused by wind. To reach a proper Chinese medical diagnosis for arthritis, differentiation based on the individual is always important.

Menstrual Disorders

Clinical manifestations

Irregular menstrual cycle. Dull or sharp pain with cold sensation in the lower abdomen or in the back during menstruation. The symptoms become worse when the patient is exposed to cold in the environment and are relieved by warmth, such as by applying a warm heating pad to the lower abdomen. The menstrual blood is usually dark and thick, and contains purple or black clots.

Key points: See Fig. 5-11 (p. 84).

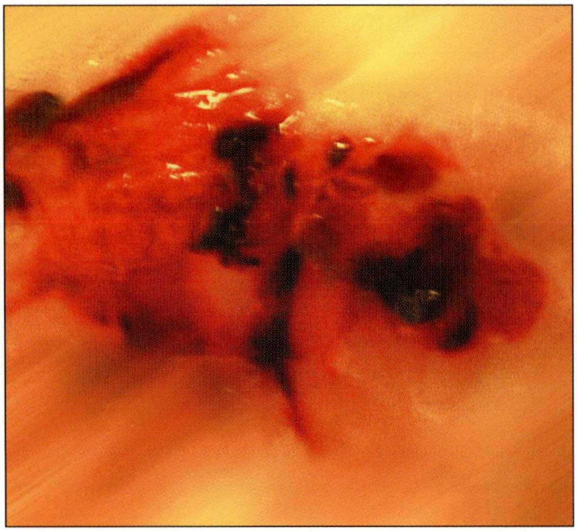

Fig. 5-11: *Dysmenorrhea*
Dark, sticky menstrual blood discharge, with purple clots

Pathological process

Dark clots in the menstrual blood are a manifestation of blood stasis in the Penetrating and Conception vessels (*chòng mài* 冲脉 and *rèn mài* 任脉) as well as in the uterus. A cold sensation indicates the presence of pathogenic cold. A sticky, thick blood discharge is due to pathogenic cold deeply invading the vessels, which slows down the circulation of blood. Cold also freezes or congeals the blood, leading to blood stasis, which results in the blood discharge becoming dark with purple clots. Pain in the lower abdomen (dysmenorrhea) is caused by blood stasis obstructing the vessels.

Because the yang qi is inhibited by pathogenic cold, this encourages the development of interior coldness, impairing the warmth provided to the vessels and uterus. Menstrual bleeding worsens the interior cold in the lower burner, leading to coldness, which can be relieved by the application of warmth, in the lower abdomen or back during menstruation. The poor circulation of qi and blood in the Penetrating and Conception vessels results in the irregular menstrual cycle.

Diagnosis

Cold blood pattern with pathogenic cold constricting the uterus (as well as the Penetrating and Conception vessels)

Lower abdominal pain indicates involvement of the uterus while the symptoms of pain with cold, intolerence of cold, and the relief provided by warmth indicate a cold pattern. Irregular menstruation reflects a disturbance of the blood and qi circulation in the Penetrating and Conception vessels and also in the uterus. The sticky, dark, and clotted menstrual blood indicates blood stasis. The blood stasis in the vessels and uterus resulting from pathogenic cold is proof that this is a pattern of cold blood.

Differential diagnosis

Cold blood patterns can be divided into two types: in the first, pathogenic cold constricts the channels and collaterals (or congeals blood in the channels and collaterals); and in the second, pathogenic cold constricts the uterus (as well as the Penetrating and Conception vessels). The pathogenic cold can be external, that is, an invasion of external pathogenic cold from the environment, or internal, that is, interior cold resulting from damage to the yang qi in the body.

Symptoms of the first pattern usually appear in the extremities, as the channels and collaterals are located in the body surface, and, compared with the trunk, the channels and collaterals of the limbs have relatively weak yang qi and a more limited ability to repel pathogenic factors. They are thus more readily affected by pathogenic cold that results in a disorder, such as pathogenic cold constricting the channels and collaterals. Examples are described in the first four sections of this chapter.

The other type of cold blood pattern, seen in this case, is one of pathogenic cold constricting the uterus, which can be explained by the physiological characteristics of the Penetrating and Conception vessels and the uterus. The Conception vessel is the sea of the yin channels and collaterals and the Penetrating vessel is the sea of the blood. The uterus, therefore, is a *fǔ* 腑 organ rich in yin and blood. Compared with the channels and organs which are rich in yang and qi, those that are rich in yin and blood are more readily affected by external or internal pathological coldness that leads to disease.

It is important to understand the differentiation of menstrual disorders caused by patterns of cold blood or patterns of blood stasis, because similar features in the color and texture of menstrual blood are present in both. The key to distinguishing between them is that patients with cold blood patterns have symptoms characterized by cold—such as a pale appearance with cold extremities or pain in the lower abdomen with a cold sensation and a desire for warmth—which are absent in patterns of blood stasis.

Dark Purple Tongue with a Moist Surface

A typical manifestation of a cold blood pattern is a dark purple or blue-purple tongue with a moist surface. (For more information, see Ch. 8 on tongue diagnosis.)

Summary

Table 5-1: *Key diagnostic points for patterns of cold blood*

Cause of Symptoms	Symptoms (Images)	Examples of Diseases and Symptoms
Pathogenic cold congeals the blood in the channels	Blue-purple or white skin on the limbs; symptoms worsen with cold (Figs. 5-1 to 5-5)	Peripheral vascular disease (e.g., Raynaud's syndrome, livedo reticularis), poor circulation (e.g., shock)
Obstruction of channels	Numbness in the limbs, necrosis and a sloughing off of the gangrenous tissue (Figs. 5-6 to 5-9)	Neuropathy (e.g., diabetic neuropathy), vascular disease (e.g., peripheral artery disease, diabetic foot, thromboangiitis obliterans)
Obstruction of yang qi	Pain with cold sensation in the hands, feet, chest, or abdomen; desire for warmth (Figs. 5-1 to 5-10)	Vascular disease (e.g., peripheral artery disease, coronary artery disease), pain (e.g., headache, arthritis)
Pathogenic cold constricts the channels and collaterals	Pain with cold, stiffness, and loss of function in joints, or deformity (Fig. 5-10)	Arthritis (e.g., rheumatoid arthritis, osteoarthritis gout, ankylosing spondylitis)
Pathogenic cold constricts the uterus	Cold and pain in the lower abdomen, prolonged menstrual cycle, dark purple clotted menstrual blood (Fig. 5-11)	Menstrual problems (e.g., irregular periods, secondary amenorrhea, dysmenorrhea, endometriosis, infertility)
Tongue and pulse	Dark purple tongue with white, moist coating; deep and slow or wiry and tight pulse (Figs. 8-7 to 8-10)	

Acupuncture point selection principles:

Tonify and warm the Kidney yang

Point selection:

CV-4, GV-4, BL-23, KI-3, BL-17

Manipulation method:

Warming and reinforcing method

Point selection for complications:

- For cold extremities: LI-4, TB-2, M-LE-8
- For numbness and cold in the hands or feet: SP-6, KI-2
- For cold sensation and pain in the lower abdomen and abnormal menstruation: CV-6, KI-13

Moxibustion is the fundamental method of treatment for cold blood patterns. Depending on the clinical situation, the moxa-stick, warming-needle method or moxa-box is chosen.

Table 5-2: *Acupuncture treatment*

<table>
<tr><th>Points</th><th>Point Explanation</th><th>Point Combinations</th></tr>
<tr><td>CV-4</td><td>The meeting point of the Conception vessel and the three leg yin channels. Serves to tonify the Kidney and strengthen basal qi.</td><td rowspan="2">CV-4 and GV-4 are an important point combination for tonifying the qi and yang of the body and strengthening the essential energy and source qi.</td></tr>
<tr><td>GV-4</td><td>Used to strengthen source qi and reinforce the Kidney yang, as the Kidney yang and qi are the root of the yang and qi for the entire body.</td></tr>
<tr><td>BL-23</td><td>The associated point of the back with the Kidney. Can regulate and strengthen the Kidney yang and qi.</td><td rowspan="2">The associated point of the back for the Kidney is combined with the source point of the Kidney channel. Moxibustion should be used on these points to warm and promote the qi and yang in the lower burner.</td></tr>
<tr><td>KI-3</td><td>The source point of the Kidney. It nourishes Kidney yin and tonifies the Kidney yang and can be used in treating deficiency of both Kidney yin and yang.</td></tr>
<tr><td>BL-17</td><td>The influential point of the blood. It can regulate the function of the blood and can also be used to nourish the blood of the body. Furthermore, it improves and harmonizes the activities of the Stomach and Spleen.</td><td></td></tr>
</table>

Treatment principle:

Warm the channels and Kidney and expel the pathogenic cold from blood level

Table 5-3: *Treatment with herbal formulas*

HERB AND DOSAGE	FLAVORS AND NATURE	ASSOCIATED CHANNELS	FORMULA ANALYSIS

■ **Tangkuei Decoction for Frigid Missing Extremities** *(dāng guī sì nì tāng)*

FOR A PATTERN OF PATHOGENIC COLD CONGEALING BLOOD AND CONSTRICTING THE CHANNELS AND COLLATERALS

HERB AND DOSAGE	FLAVORS AND NATURE	ASSOCIATED CHANNELS	FORMULA ANALYSIS
Angelicae sinensis Radix *(dāng guī)*, 12g	Sweet, acrid, and warm	Liver and Heart	Nourish the blood and regulate the circulation of blood
Paeoniae Radix *(sháo yào)*, 9g	Bitter and slightly cold	Liver and Spleen	
Cinnamomi Ramulus *(guì zhī)*, 9g	Acrid and warm	Heart, Lung, and Bladder	Expel pathogenic cold from blood level and warm the channels to remove obstructions
Asari Radix et Rhizoma *(xì xīn)*, 1.5g	Acrid and warm	Lung and Kidney	
Tetrapanacis Medulla *(tōng cǎo)*, 3g	Sweet, bland and slightly cold	Lung and Stomach	
Jujubae Fructus *(dà zǎo)*, 8 pieces	Sweet and warm	Spleen and Stomach	Tonify the Spleen to protect the antipathogenic factors
Glycyrrhizae Radix *(gān cǎo)*, 5g	Sweet and neutral	Heart, Lung, Spleen, and Stomach	

Generating and Transforming Decoction *(shēng huà tāng)*

FOR A PATTERN OF PATHOGENIC COLD CONSTRICTING THE UTERUS, PENETRATING AND CONCEPTION VESSELS

HERB AND DOSAGE	FLAVORS AND NATURE	ASSOCIATED CHANNELS	FORMULA ANALYSIS
Angelicae sinensis Radix *(dāng guī)*, 25g	Sweet, acrid, and warm	Liver and Heart	Nourish the blood and regulate the circulation of blood and the menstrual period
Chuanxiong Rhizoma *(chuān xiōng)*, 9g	Acrid and warm	Liver and Gallbladder	
Persicae Semen *(táo rén)*, 6g	Bitter and neutral	Heart and Liver	
Zingiberis Rhizoma preparata *(páo jiāng)*, 2g	Bitter and warm	Spleen and Liver	These herbs expel pathogenic cold from the blood level, warm the channels to remove the obstruction, alleviate pain
Cinnamomi Cortex *(ròu guì)*, 3g	Acrid and warm	Kidney, Spleen, Heart, and Liver	
Glycyrrhizae Radix *(gān cǎo)*, 2g	Sweet and neutral	Heart, Lung, Spleen, and Stomach	Tonifies the Spleen to protect the antipathogenic factor

CHAPTER 6

Blood Stasis Patterns and Secondary Blood Stasis Patterns Caused by Qi Stagnation or Qi Deficiency

Blue Lips

Clinical manifestations

Cyanosis (bluish discoloration of the skin and mucous membranes), most noticeably in the lips and fingernails

Key points: See Figs. 6-1 through 6-4 (pp. 92-93).

Pathological process

Blood stasis in Chinese medicine can imply poor blood circulation, but not necessarily the presence of blood clots or thrombosis (or embolism), nor that the circulation has come to a complete stop.

The lips, which are covered by thin skin and mucous membranes, allow the blood vessels underneath to appear through their surface. A rich supply of blood gives them a normal light red coloration. For patients with blood stasis, a low level of oxygen in the blood due to poor circulation results in the bluish color of cyanosis present in the skin and membranes.

According to Chinese medicine, the qi provides the energy to enable the flow of blood. It therefore follows that disorders of the qi commonly result in blood stasis. There are two types of qi disorders that lead to this condition of blood stasis: qi stagnation and qi deficiency.

In the case of qi stagnation, obstruction of qi circulation disrupts the flow of blood, giving the patient the characteristic blue appearance of cyanosis, as well as dark skin. In the case of qi deficiency, which may be brought about either by reduced production

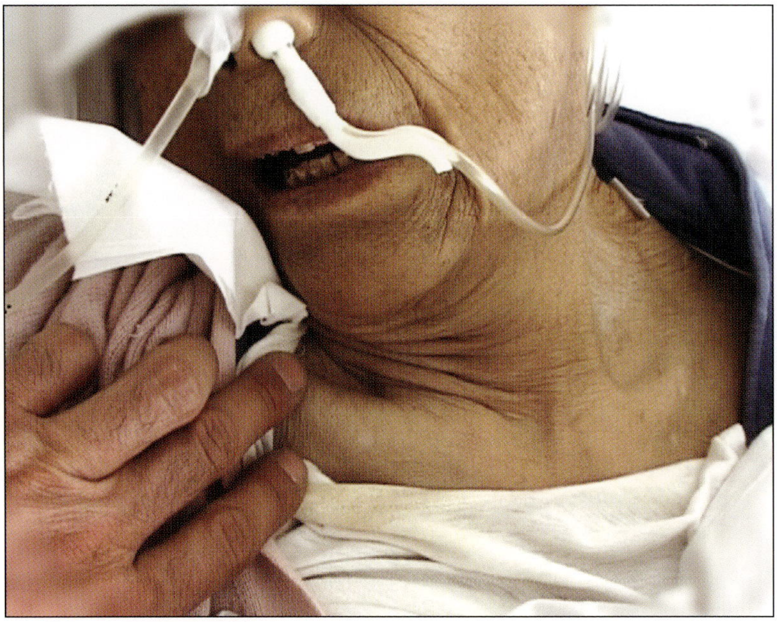

Fig. 6-1: *Kidney failure with uremia*

The patient is comatose. Note the cyanosis of the lips.

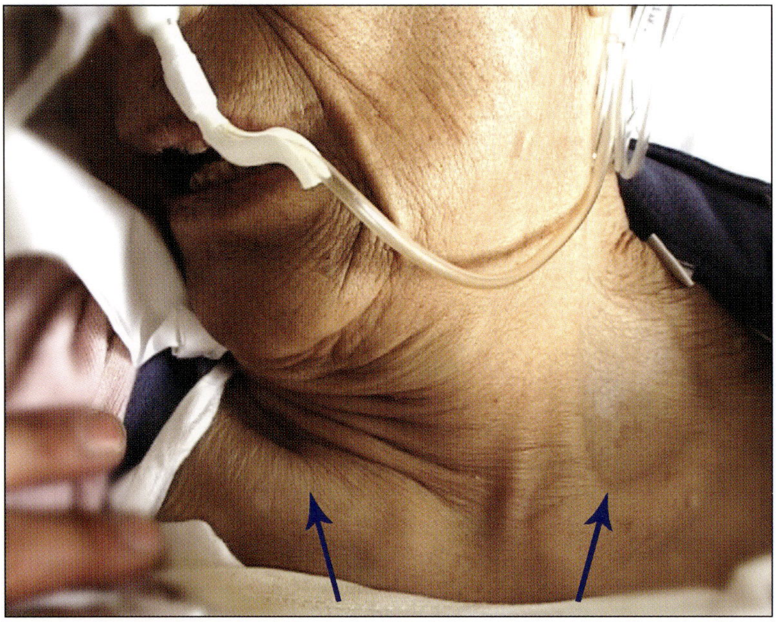

Fig. 6-2: *Same patient as above*

The patient is demonstrating breathlessness (dyspnea). As the patient inhales, the muscles in her neck and shoulders can be observed to contract. She also has a noticeable abnormality of skin color and appearance. Her skin is grey, bloodless, and lusterless; it is also withered and sallow, resulting from severe kidney failure and dehydration.

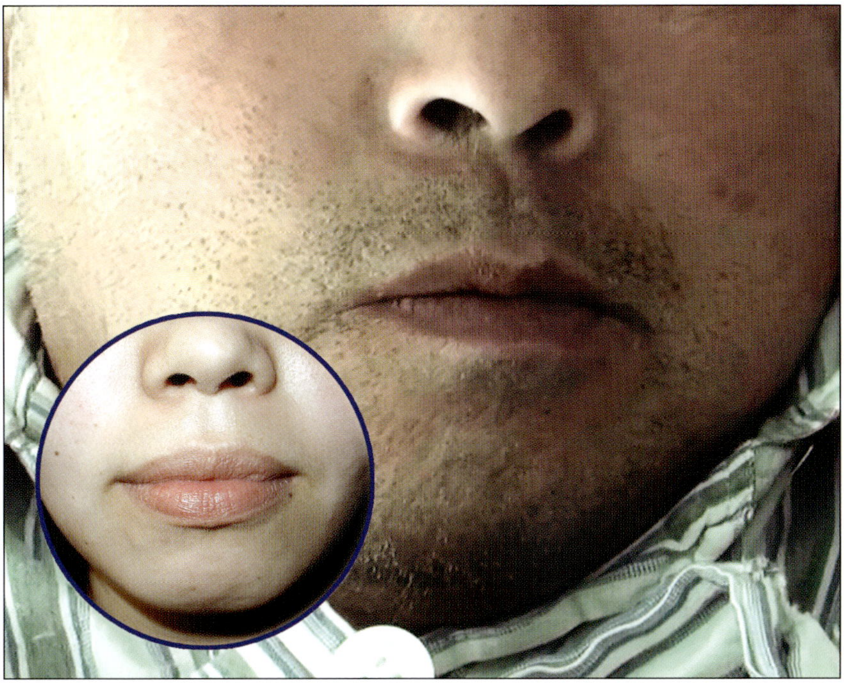

Fig. 6-3: *Chronic cor pulmonale*

This photo shows cyanosis characterized by bluish discoloration of the lips, as well as dark and lusterless skin, compared to a person with normal lips (inset).

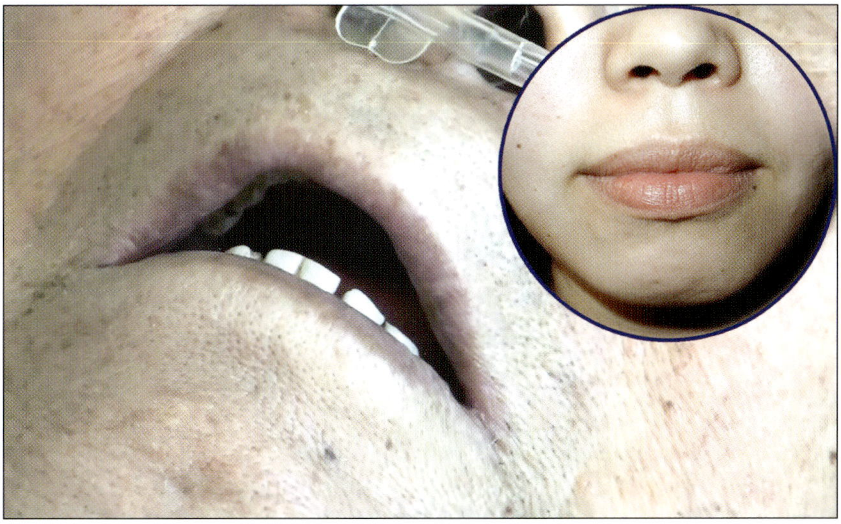

Fig. 6-4: *Cerebrovascular disease (ischemic stroke)*

This photo shows that the patient is breathless and comatose and that the lips and skin are blue-purple, dusky, and lusterless. He is compared to a person with normal lips (inset) that are light red in color, soft, moist, and lustrous.

or by increased consumption, cyanosis is always accompanied by shortness of breath and exhaustion or fatigue.

Diagnosis

Blood stasis with poor circulation of blood

Cyanosis is a sign of poor blood circulation in the channels and collaterals. This means that the three patients shown above all have blood stasis. Those shown in Figs. 6-1 and 6-4 both share a secondary blood stasis pattern caused by qi deficiency. Unconsciousness indicates severe damage to the antipathogenic factors. Difficulty in breathing (dyspnea) indicates Lung qi deficiency. The signs of bloodless, withered, sallow skin and general emaciation suggest consumption of the qi.

The patient shown in Fig. 6-3 suffers from a secondary blood stasis pattern caused by qi stagnation. He has difficulty breathing but does not feel a shortness of breath. He is not emaciated but does have an obvious cyanosis along with a dark and lusterless complexion, indicating that the disorder is qi stagnation rather than qi deficiency.

Differential diagnosis

A pattern of blood stasis can be either a primary condition or a secondary condition caused by a qi disorder. If the latter, one must search for the underlying cause of the blood stasis. In this group of patients, blood stasis results from either qi deficiency or stagnation. Regardless of the cause, the symptoms of blood stasis are virtually the same. The key point for differentiation is to look for evidence of qi deficiency or qi stagnation.

In addition to the differentiations noted above, typical symptoms of qi deficiency patterns are a lack of energy such as lassitude, weak voice, poor appetite, or diarrhea. A reduced capacity for exercise and shortness of breath that worsens during physical activity are also common symptoms of qi deficiency. In patterns of qi stagnation there is obstruction of qi activity in the body; typical symptoms include a feeling of tightness in the chest, distention in the costal regions, and harsh wheezing with a suffocating sensation.

Brown or Purple Skin

Clinical manifestations

Brown or purple spots with rough and dry skin

Key points: See Figs. 6-5 and 6-6 (p. 95).

Pathological process

Brown or purple skin is an early manifestation of poor circulation of blood in the channels and collaterals. The slowing down and then accumulation of blood in the lo-

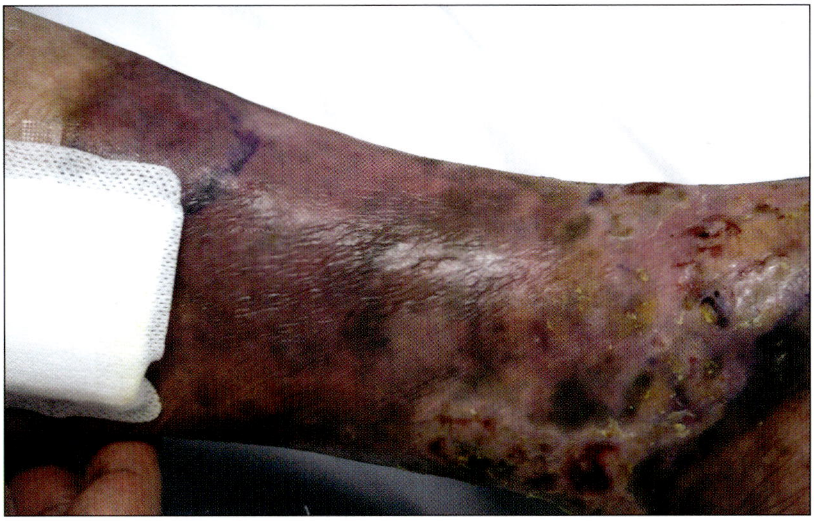

Fig. 6-5: *Stasis dermatitis with infection*

The skin of the lower leg has became dark brown or purple in color. There are some suppurating skin ulcers on the surface. The patient complains of extreme tenderness.

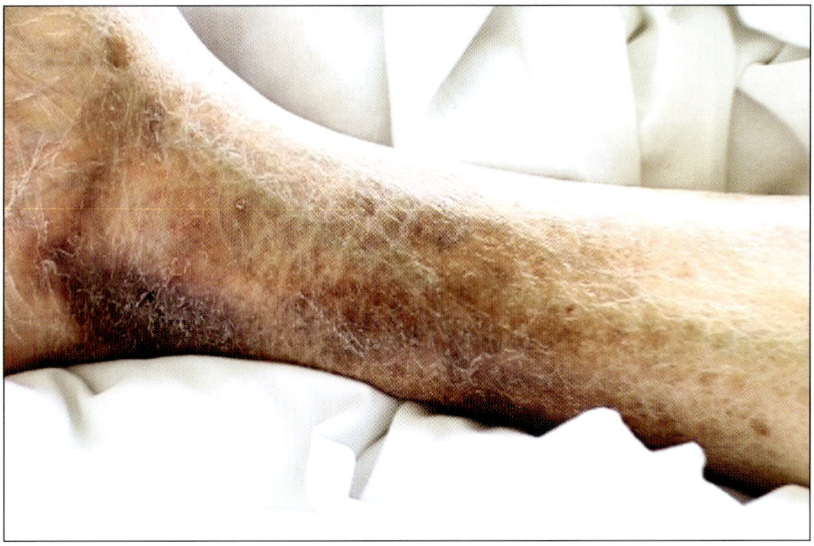

Fig. 6-6: *Diabetes, skin spots*

Dark brown spots appear on the back of the ankle. The dark area of skin is lusterless, rough, dry, and scaly.

cal collaterals results in blood stasis; dark brown spots then appear. The obstruction of collaterals due to blood stasis leads to the failure of yang qi to reach the local skin, which thereupon becomes lusterless. The obstruction of the collaterals also prevents the blood from reaching and nourishing the local skin, causing the skin to become dry, rough, and scaly. Skin ulcers are characteristic of dampness.

Diagnosis

Blood stasis in the local collaterals

Localized discoloration of the skin indicates a superficial disorder in which only the collaterals are affected. The dryness, roughness, and scaly skin around the area of the foot and ankle in this case (Fig. 6-6) indicates that there is poor blood circulation, but it has not reached a serious stage: the blood stasis is not severe. In Fig. 6-5, suppurating skin ulcers on the surface and tenderness indicate an obstruction of the channels caused by an invasion of dampness, which may be the reason for the blood stasis in this case.

Differential diagnosis

The brown or purple skin (muddy-brown pigmentation) shown in Fig. 6-6 is the most common sign of blood stasis. It can be observed in any part of the body, usually on the legs. It typically indicates a superficial obstruction in the collaterals, if there are no other disorders.

Blackened Skin

Clinical manifestations

Tan or black spots and dry, thickening, rough or cracked skin

Key points: See Figs. 6-7 and 6-8 (p. 97).

Pathological process

Blackened skin is a manifestation of prolonged blood stasis.

The accumulation of blood in the channels and collaterals has resulted in the skin first turning brown and then black, as the blocked circulation in the channels has not improved for a long period of time. The obstruction leads to a failure of the yang qi to reach the surface of the body and thus the skin becomes lusterless. Malnourishment of the skin results in its dry, rough, and cracked appearance, which results from blood being unable to circulate through the blocked channels and collaterals. The pathological processes here are similar to those in the previous cases. The differences will be discussed later.

Diagnosis

Blood stasis in the channels and collaterals

In contrast to the brown or purple skin mentioned in the previous cases, the black skin here indicates that the history of the disorder is much longer and that blood stasis is persistantly blocking the channels and collaterals. The rough and cracked skin reflects malnourishment of the skin. (See the following case for more details.)

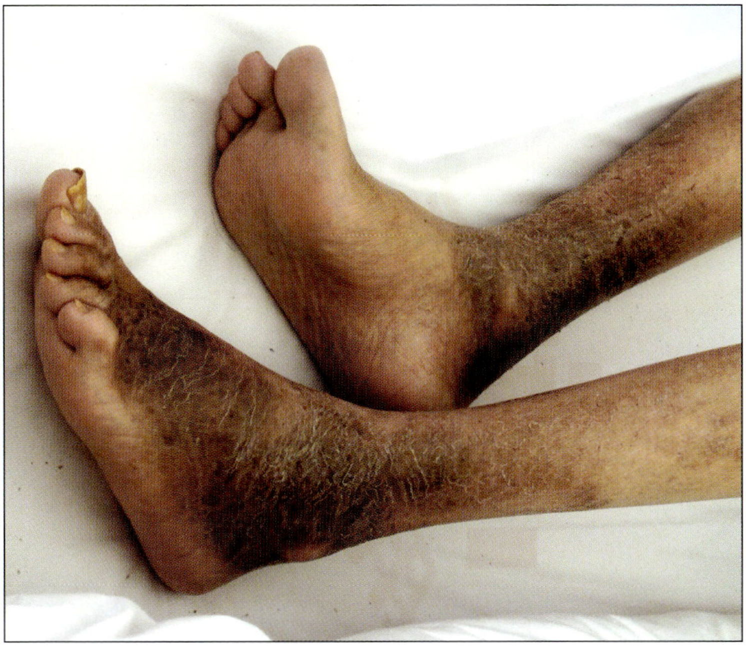

Fig. 6-7: *Diabetes, skin spots*

Cracked, dark brown, and black skin appears on the lower legs and feet.

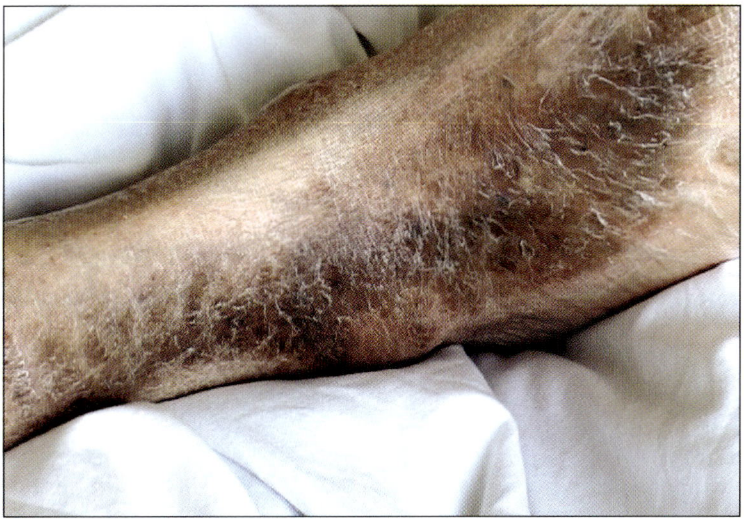

Fig. 6-8: *Diabetes, skin spots*

The skin spots on the right lower limb are black in color and the skin itself is dry, rough, lusterless, and cracked.

Differential diagnosis

In the clinic, blackened skin is usually associated with a more serious stage in a disorder for which discoloration of the skin is a symptom. In patterns of blood stasis, the darker the color, the more severe and prolonged the obstruction in the channels and collaterals.

A patient with a pattern of cold blood can also have black skin. This is due to the constant constriction and blockage of the circulation of blood in the channels and collaterals by cold; if not relieved, it presents a much more serious problem with potentially severe consequences. (See Ch. 5 on patterns of cold blood for more details.)

Rough and Scaly Skin

Clinical manifestations

The color of the skin can be brown, purple, or black. Darkened areas can become dry, rough, thick or scaly, and can crack and peel.

Key points: See Figs. 6-9 through 6-11 (below and p. 99).

Pathological process

Rough and scaly skin is a manifestation of poor skin nourishment. It can be evidence of a skin condition or a cutaneous sign associated with systemic disease. According to Chinese medicine, blood pertains to yin and is circulated by the yang qi, the energy within the body, so that it is distributed all around the body, nourishing and moistening the organs and the skin. If blood stasis causes an obstruction of the channels and collaterals, the qi and blood cannot reach the skin, which leads to skin disorders. Because the skin is deprived of its nourishment by the blood and yang qi, it loses its normal color and luster. Blood stasis affects the channels and collaterals of the body

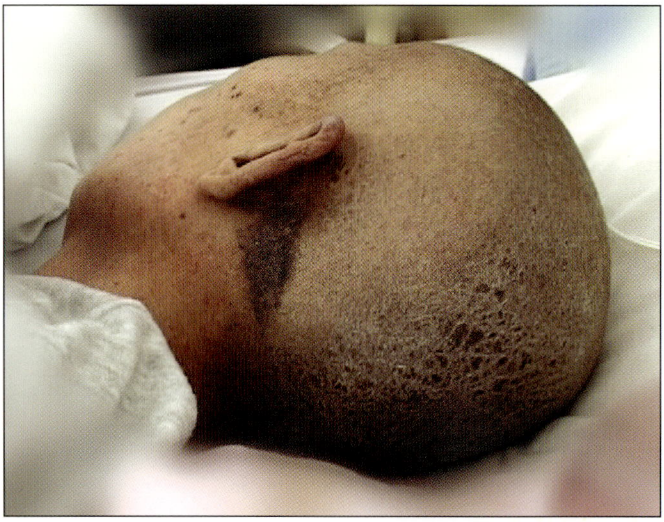

Fig. 6-9: *Brain tumor*

Darkening and thickening of the skin appears on the back of the head. The scaly patches are dry, rough, slightly raised, and cracked.

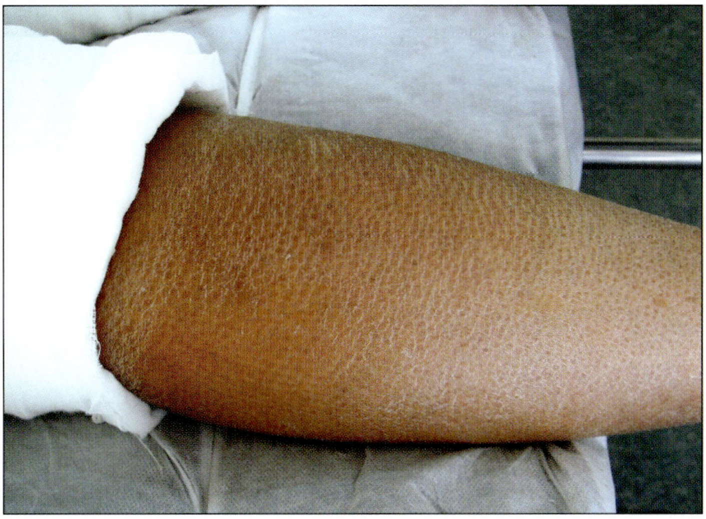

Fig. 6-10: *Bone fracture*
Brown, scar-like patches appear on the leg.

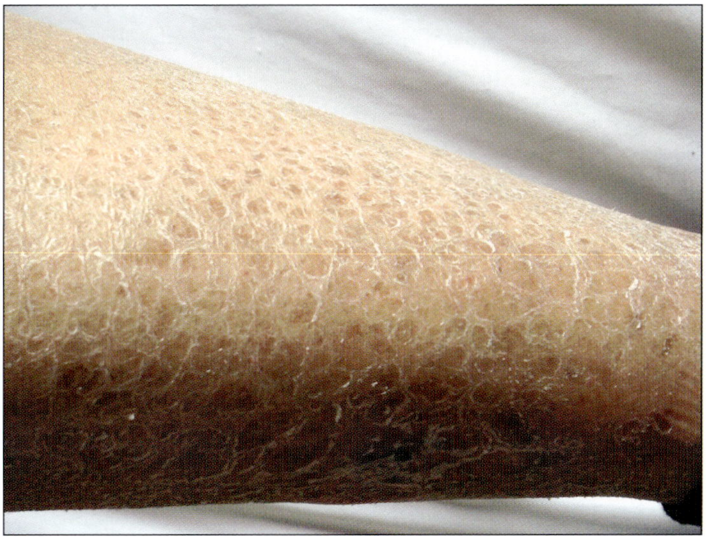

Fig. 6-11: *Diabetic dermopathy*
Dark brown and scaly patches appear on the leg, without pain or itchiness.

that supply the skin with blood as well as other body fluids. Deprived of moisture, the skin becomes dry, thick, and rough. After a period of time, malnourishment of the skin due to blood stasis in the channels and collaterals leads to poor elasticity and cracking of the skin.

Diagnosis

Blood stasis with malnourishment of the skin

The skin disorders described here involve the alteration of skin color, loss of skin luster, and changes in skin texture associated with organ disorders. Among these manifestations, the darkened skin color indicates blood stasis, the lusterlessness of the skin indicates an obstruction of yang qi, and changes in the texture, such as rough and thickened skin, poor elasticity, or cracked skin, indicate an obstruction of the channels and collaterals over a long period of time.

Differential diagnosis

Rough and scaly skin (*jī fū jiă cuò* 肌肤甲错) represents a long history of blood stasis, often associated with chronic systemic diseases or malignant conditions (like cachexia). Clinically, the changes can be seen on any part of the body but are more likely found on the lower limbs.

The basic pathological process in rough and scaly skin is blood stasis, which usually develops as a result of one of the following: external pathogenic factors that lead to an obstruction in the channels and collaterals; an obstruction of qi activity that causes qi stagnation leading to blood stasis; or diminished strength of circulation that causes qi deficiency leading to blood stasis. This is why, when approaching a patient with blood stasis, it is necessary to ascertain if there is an underlying cause. It is also important to realize that most skin conditions mentioned in this book, as in the clinic, are a manifestation of a disease of the internal organ systems; that is, it is often a symptom of a disease rather than the disease itself.

Bruises

Clinical manifestations

The skin and surrounding region become blue or purple, tender, and swollen following an injury.

Key points: See Figs. 6-12 and 6-13 (p. 101).

Pathological process

Bruises that occur after an injury indicate subcutaneous bleeding.

The impact of the injury does not damage the skin, but breaks the walls of the blood vessels, or, according to Chinese medicine, injures the channels and collaterals, causing the blood to escape from the vessels and accumulate under the skin (blood stasis), which results in bruises and swelling. An acute injury will not cause malnourishment of the skin, as the history of such an injury is normally short, and thus the elasticity and texture of the skin does not change. Because there is blood stasis locally and the collaterals are obstructed, the pain is very severe.

Diagnosis

Injury causing blood stasis

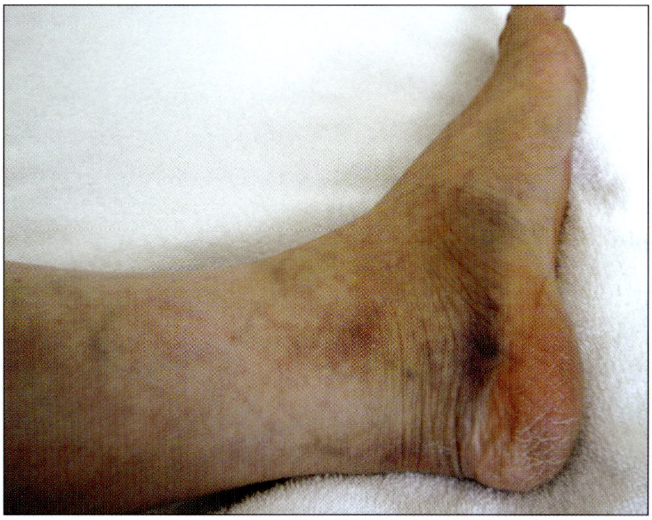

Fig. 6-12: *Ankle injury*

A large purple bruise can be seen on the inner side of the ankle following an injury and subcutaneous hemorrhage. The color of the bruise does not change with pressure. There is obvious local tissue elevation and hematoma around the ankle, which has lost its normal appearance.

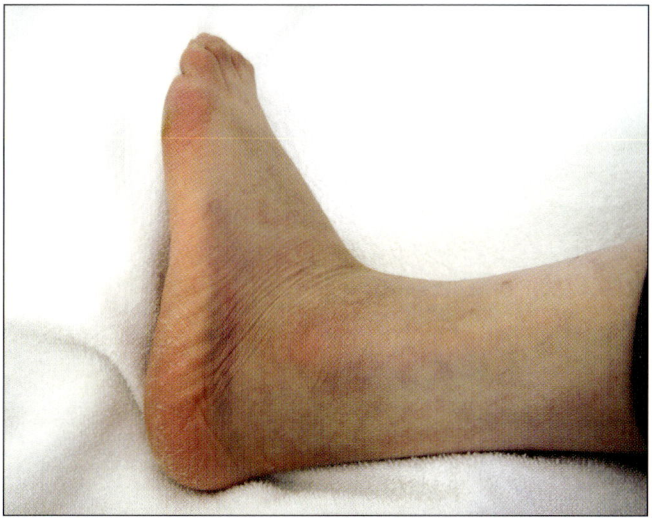

Fig. 6-13: *Same patient, ankle injury*

Light purple bruise on the lateral section of the same ankle. The elasticity and texture of the skin has not changed very much.

The history of injury and the symptoms of pain and swelling indicate an injury to and obstruction of the local channels and collaterals. Bruises which are blue or purple and then turn black indicate that blood stasis has accumulated locally. The skin on the remainder of the leg has normal luster and moisture, indicating that the injury in this case is localized.

Differential diagnosis

In this particular case, there is a definite history of injury and therefore there is no need to consider other possible diagnoses. Bruises generally indicate that there is hemorrhaging under the skin, which can extend over a large or small area. The appearance of the bruise is determined by the extent and severity of the injury.

Vascular Spider (Spider Angioma)

Clinical manifestations

Small red dots on the face, upper part of the trunk, and hands. Pressing on the dots causes the redness to disappear briefly. Distention and pain in the costal regions are common symptoms.

Key points: See Figs. 6-14 through 6-18 (pp. 103-105).

Pathological process

Vascular spiders are particular manifestations of blood stasis in the Liver.

According to Chinese medicine, the qi is the governor of the blood which means that it provides the energy to circulate the blood. The Liver is responsible for the free-flowing of qi (or the qi dynamic) and therefore regulates the qi activity of the entire body. If the Liver qi functions normally and the qi moves smoothly throughout the body, normal circulation of qi and blood will occur.

Liver dysfunction will affect the free-flowing of the qi (or the qi dynamic), causing qi stagnation and thus a slowing of the blood flow, which creates blood stasis in the organs as well as in the surface of the body. The blood stasis causes localized accumulation of blood in the channels and collaterals, and thus small red dots or spider angiomas appear. An increase of blood in the collaterals, known as congestion, does not cause a hemorrhage because the blood remains in the collaterals, which have not suffered any injury, and is still being circulated. This explains why, when pressure is applied to the spot, the red or purple areas disappear, then reappear when the pressure is released.

Diagnosis

Secondary blood stasis caused by qi stagnation

Distention and pain in the costal regions indicate a stagnation of Liver qi. Small red spots (vascular spiders) in the skin indicate blood stasis. Visible blood vessels that radiate from the center indicate that the accumulation of blood in the collaterals is close to the body surface. The color of the spots in the skin, which disappears with pressure

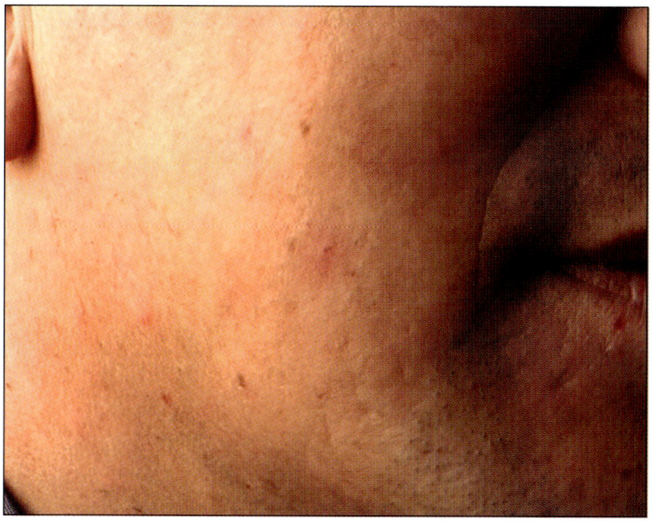

Fig. 6-14: *Cirrhosis (hepatic cirrhosis)*

Vascular spider on the cheek. There is a small purple dot (dilated arteriole) in the center with reddish extensions (telangiectasias) radiating from the center, resembling a spider's legs.

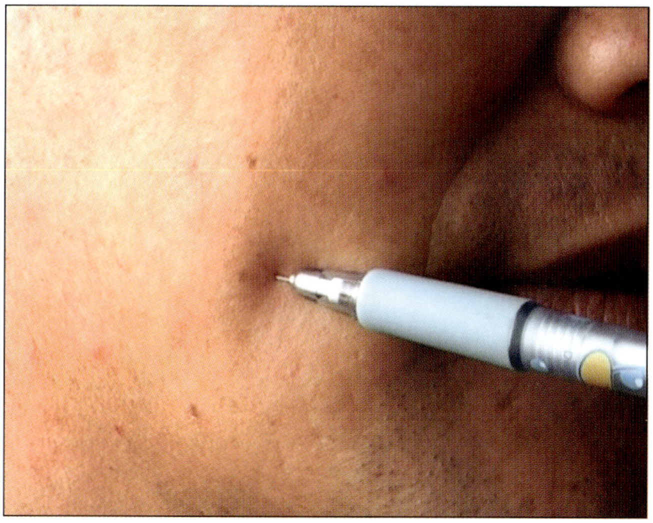

Fig. 6-15: *Application of pressure to the vascular spider*

and reappears when the pressure is released, indicates that the blood is still circulating in the collaterals and that there is neither injury to the vessels nor hemorrhaging.

Differential diagnosis

Red or purple spots on the skin with the characteristics described above are not a common manifestation of blood stasis patterns, but should they appear, they can

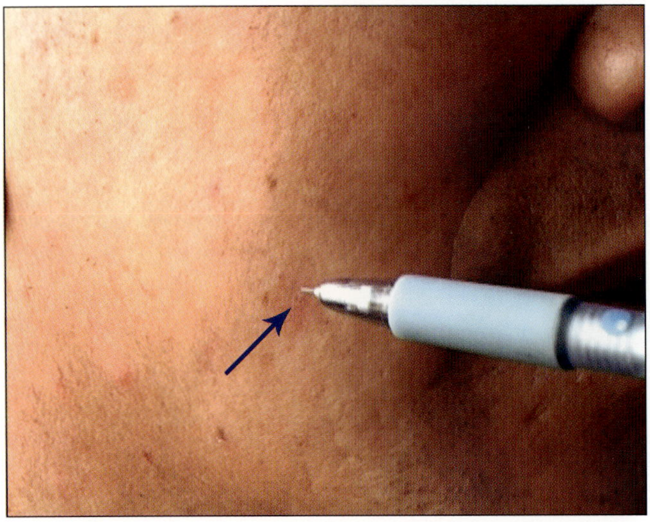

Fig. 6-16: *Purple outlines of the vascular spider disappear*

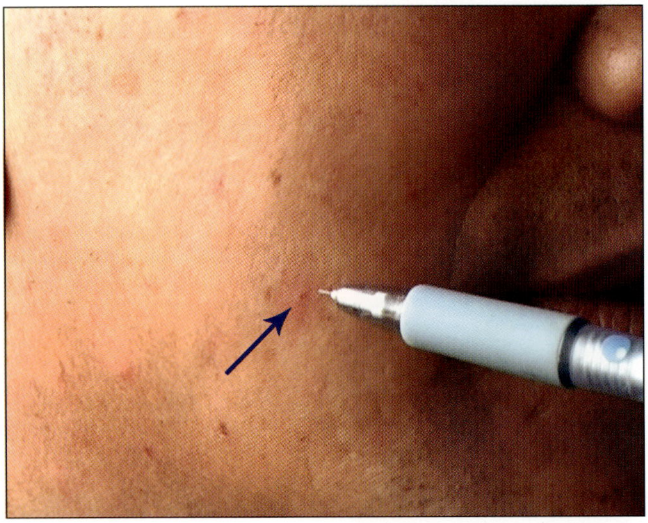

Fig. 6-17: *Reappearance of the purple outlines when pressure is released*

support a diagnosis of blood stasis—especially blood stasis caused by qi stagnation.

Some of these characteristics are similar to those of a skin rash. Although skin rashes often occur in hot blood patterns, they do not do so in patterns of blood stasis. (See Ch. 4 for more details on hot blood patterns.)

In conventional medicine, spider angiomas (vascular spiders) often appear when a patient has a hepatic disease. According to Chinese medicine, such a patient often suffers from patterns of qi stagnation and blood stasis.

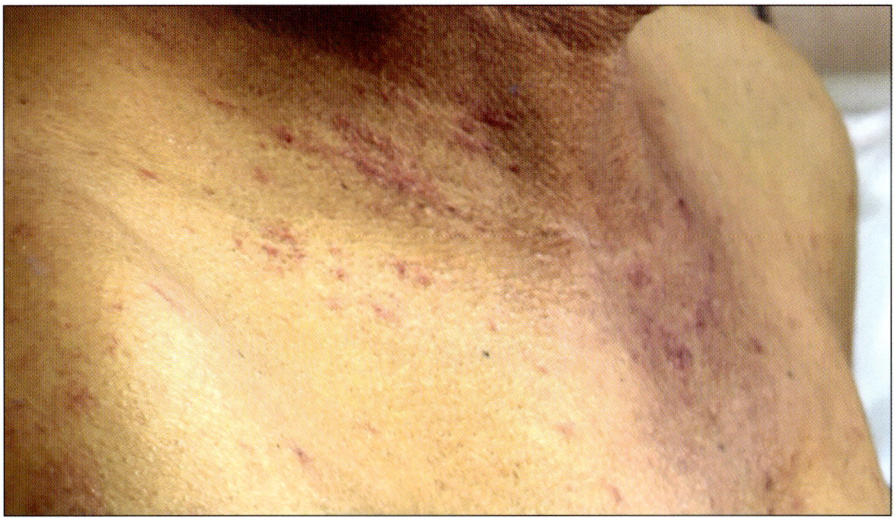

Fig. 6-18: *Another patient with cirrhosis (hepatic cirrhosis)*
There are several red spots (vascular spiders) visible on the upper part of the patient's trunk.

Blood Clots

Clinical manifestations

Hemorrhages, seen as menorrhagia, hematuria, hematemesis, or melena, or as bleeding in patients with advanced cancer. The color of the blood is dark, dark purple or black, and blood clots are present. The blood clots are most commonly encountered during heavy menstrual periods. The menstrual blood can be red or dark and thick, with purple or black clots. Patients also complain of prolonged or painful menstrual periods.

Key points: See Fig. 6-19 (p. 106).

Masses

Clinical manifestations

A firm, irregular, or lumpy abdominal mass can be detected on physical examination. Patients often suffer from abdominal distention or pain, fatigue, emaciation, or a severe loss of weight.

Key points: See Figs. 6-20 through 6-22 (pp. 106-107).

Pathological process

One form of abdominal mass is blood stasis in the organs of the abdominal cavity. In Chinese medicine, the classical explanation for the cause of a mass is a severe block-

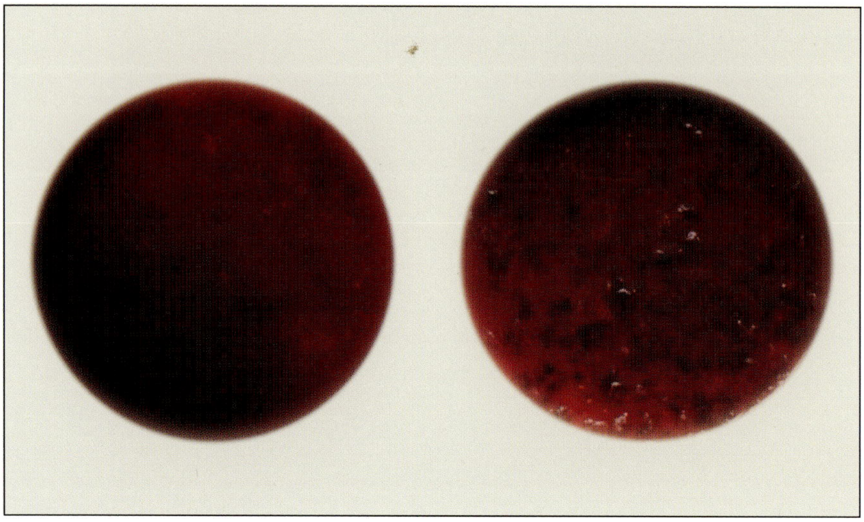

Fig. 6-19: *Irregular periods*

A few dark purple or black clots can be seen in the dark red, thick menstrual blood. The patient also complains of sharp lower abdominal pain and dull back pain, which begin several days before and last until after the first few days of her period. (See Ch. 7 on bleeding for more details.)

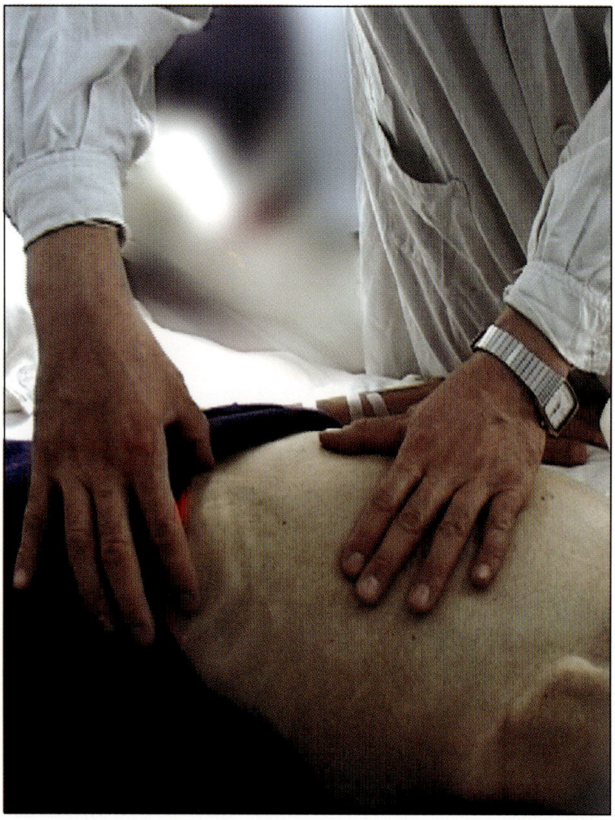

Fig. 6-20: *Advanced stage of cancer with ascites*

A large, hard, and painful growth that can be felt in the upper right quadrant of the abdomen (below the right costal margin). The size of the mass is indicated by the space between the doctor's hands. The mass is firm and fixed and is attached to deep tissues so that it cannot be easily moved. The patient also has severe weight loss.

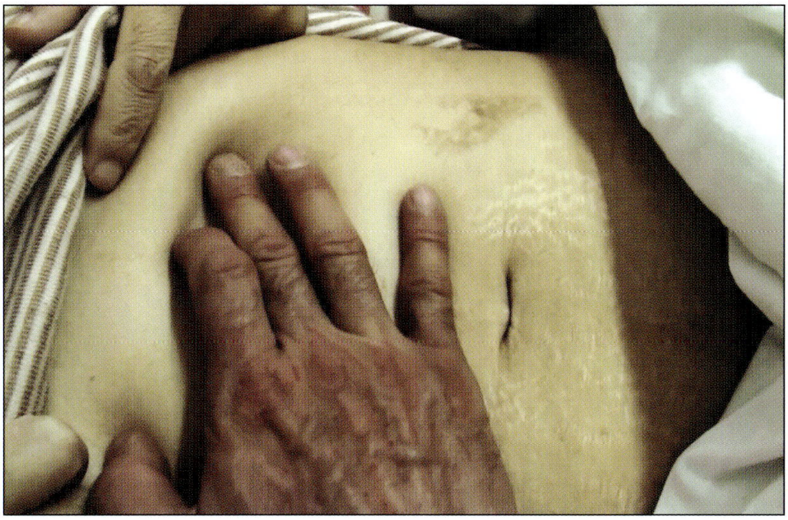

Fig. 6-21: *Hemolytic anemia with jaundice*

A noticeably enlarged spleen can be detected. The image shows the enlargement of the spleen, which can be felt below the left costal margin.

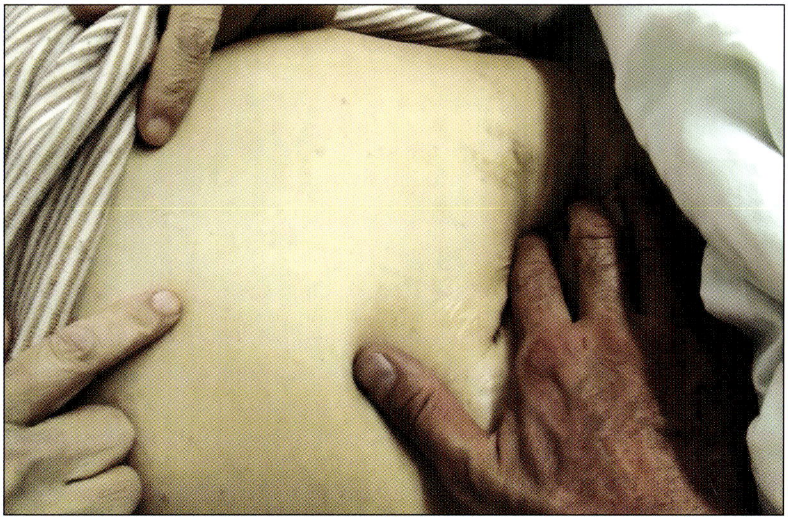

Fig. 6-22: *Same patient*

This shows the size of the spleen enlargement.

age of blood circulation. As the blood is obstructed and accumulates in the local area, masses can result. In this group of cases, blood stasis has occurred in the left or right hypochondriac region.

According to Chinese medicine, blood stasis is one of the substantial pathogenic factors. When blood stasis occurs in a certain place, it remains there, which is why a hard, irregularly-shaped mass can be detected. The mass may be attached to or can grow with deeper tissue, and so it is fixed. Blood stasis blocks the circulation of blood and qi in the channels and collaterals, causing abdominal pain that may be too tender to be palpated. The swollen abdomen is due to qi stagnation and retention of pathogenic water. (For more information, see Ch. 2 on Spleen qi deficiency.)

The pathogenic factor in this case, blood stasis, has persisted in the body for a long period of time: the qi, blood, yin, and essence have all been severely consumed, resulting in the patient's weight loss and emaciation. The yellowing of the skin (jaundice) is associated with pathogenic damp-heat, which can be either an external or internal pathogenic factor.

Diagnosis

Blood stasis and qi stagnation along with Spleen qi and Spleen yang deficiency, as well as retention of pathogenic water

The distended upper right quadrant of the abdomen and the firm mass that can be detected indicate blood stasis in the abdomen. The general enlargement of the abdomen indicates that, in addition to blood stasis, there is also stagnation of qi and retention of pathogenic water within the abdominal cavity. Severe fatigue and obvious emaciation are the result of a severe injury to the antipathogenic factors. In this case (Fig. 6-20), the pathogenic factors are strong and the antipathogenic factors have been quite weakened, so the prognosis is poor.

Differential diagnosis

Growths or masses caused by blood stasis can be seen in various parts of the body, including the abdominal cavity, the arms and legs, and also the skin or subcutaneous tissue (below the skin). No matter where the growth or tumor occurs, they all share certain characteristics:

- They are firm and fixed.
- They are irregular in shape.
- They are painful and tender to palpation.

There are other possible causes of masses found in the abdominal cavity, such as pathogenic phlegm, retention of pathogenic water, qi stagnation, retention of food, or retention of feces (fecal impaction). The location of the mass as well as its firmness, texture, and other features, and also the general symptoms, can provide clues as to the cause of the mass.

Visibly Enlarged Veins

Clinical manifestations

Enlarged veins above the surface of the skin, which can be dark purple or blue

Key points: See Figs. 6-23 through 6-26 (pp. 109-110).

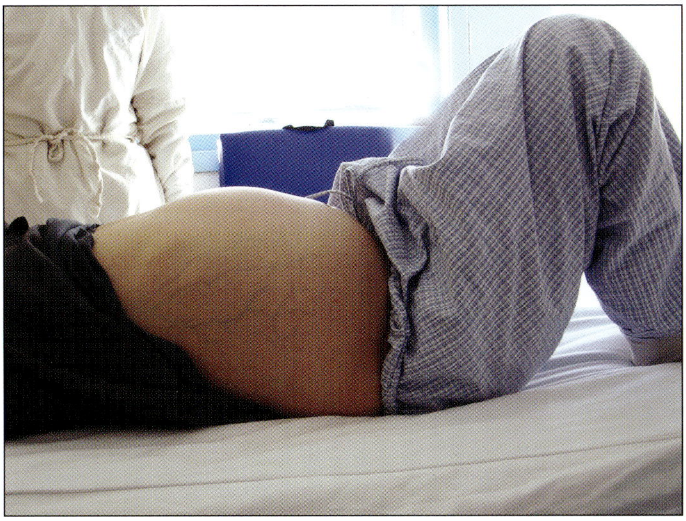

Fig. 6-23: *Alcoholic cirrhosis*

The image shows a distended and swollen abdomen and the appearance of distended and engorged veins across the abdomen.

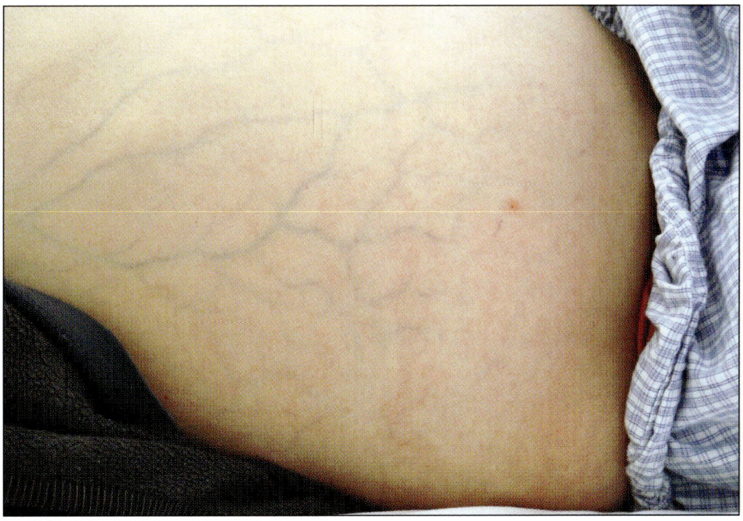

Fig. 6-24: *Same patient*

A closer view of the distended abdominal wall veins

Pathological process

In Chinese medical theory, these dilated, twisted veins above the skin are a manifestation of blood stasis in the channels and collaterals. The first patient's abdominal distention (Figs. 6-23 and 6-24) is caused by retention of pathogenic water, which is associated with a substantial pathogenic factor. A build-up of pathogenic water in the abdominal cavity (peritoneal cavity) blocks the circulation and causes the blood

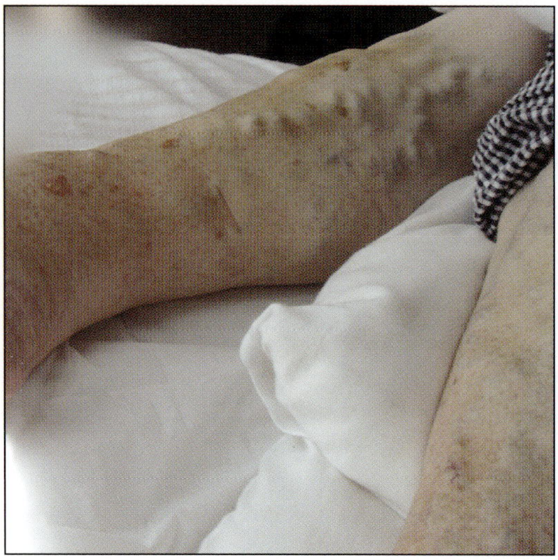

Fig. 6-25: *Varicose veins in the leg*

Enlarged blue veins, swollen and raised above the surface of the skin. They appear twisted and bulging.

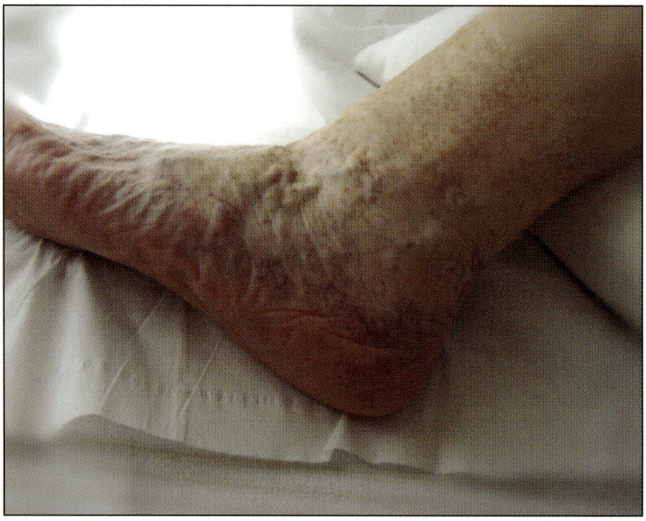

Fig. 6-26: *Same patient*

Swollen, raised, and enlarged veins around the ankle

to accumulate in the channels. This is why the enlarged veins are visible through the skin of the abdomen.

The second patient (Figs. 6-25 and 6-26) has blood stasis in the superficial collaterals of the legs and feet. Following the same pathological process discussed in this chapter, the poor circulation led to an excessive accumulation of blood in the collaterals, and the veins became twisted and bulging. Both blue and purple veins signify the presence of blood stasis.

Diagnosis

Blood stasis in the channels and collaterals

In the first case, large veins can be observed through the skin of the abdomen, indicating blood stasis in the organs. Together with retention of pathogenic water in the abdominal cavity (peritoneal cavity), this is evidence of a severe condition.

The second case is a typical example of varicose veins. The appearance of blue bulging veins on the legs indicates that the blood stasis is limited to the surface and that only the local collaterals have been affected. Without proper treatment, dark purple skin (stasis dermatitis) or skin ulcers (venous ulcers) may develop because the blood stasis may lead to malnourishment of the skin.

Differential diagnosis

Enlarged veins above the surface of the skin together with the swollen abdomen suggest the retention of substantial pathogenic factors in the body, the most common of which are pathogenic water and/or blood stasis. In this chapter, the key point is to find clinical evidence of blood stasis. (For more information about harmful water retention, see Ch. 2 on Spleen deficiency [Fig. 2-13]).

Dark Purple Tongue

A typical manifestation of blood stasis patterns on the tongue is a dark purple coloration and/or ecchymosis or spots on the surface or around the border of the tongue body and a lack of luster. (See Ch. 8 on tongue diagnosis for more details.)

Summary

Table 6-1: *Key diagnostic points for blood stasis patterns and secondary blood stasis patterns*

Cause of Symptoms	Symptoms (Images)	Examples of Diseases and Symptoms
Poor blood circulation in the mucous membranes (cyanosis)	Blue-purple lips and fingernails (Figs. 6-1 to 6-4)	Respiratory diseases (e.g., asthma, pulmonary emphysema), cardiovascular diseases (e.g., heart failure, some congenital heart diseases, chronic cor pulmonale)
Localized blood stasis	Blue-purple or black color or bruises on the skin (Figs. 6-5 to 6-8, and 6-12 to 6-13)	Injury (e.g., bruise following injury), systemic diseases (e.g., diabetic dermopathy), purpura (e.g., anaphylactoid allergic purpura, idiopathic thrombocytopenic purpura)

—continued next page

Cause of Symptoms	Symptoms (Images)	Examples of Diseases and Symptoms
Malnourishment of skin	Scaly and rough skin (Figs. 6-9 to 6-11)	Malignant conditions (e.g., cancer), cachexia (e.g., chronic infections or systemic diseases), skin conditions
Blockage of blood in the channels and collaterals	Prickling or throbbing pain, worsens with pressure	Pain (e.g., gastric ulcer, headache), injury (e.g., car crash, sports injury), thrombosis (e.g., coronary artery disease, stroke)
Blood stasis in the organs	Firm, hard, and fixed masses (Figs. 6-20 to 6-22)	Internal organ (e.g., enlarged liver or spleen), tumors (e.g., stomach or liver cancer, goiter)
Blood stasis in the vessels	Dilated, twisted veins or vascular spiders in the skin (Figs. 6-23 to 6-26, and 6-14 to 6-18)	Liver disease (e.g., hepatic cirrhosis, portal hypertension), vein problems (e.g., varicose veins in the leg, varicocele)
Blood stasis in the uterus, Penetrating and Conception vessels	Dark and thick menstrual bleeding with purple or black clots (Fig. 6-19)	Menstrual disorders (e.g., irregular or prolonged menstrual cycle, dysfunctional uterine bleeding, secondary amenorrhea, dysmenorrhoea, endometriosis)
Hemorrhage caused by blood stasis	Dark red or purple clotted blood and recurrent hemorrhaging	Hemorrhages (e.g., hematemesis or hematochezia, purpura), internal bleeding (e.g., bleeding from the liver or spleen)
Secondary blood stasis caused by qi stagnation	Distention, fullness, suffocating sensation either in chest or abdomen; irritability or hot temper (Figs. 6-3, 6-14 to 6-18, 6-20 to 6-24)	Respiratory diseases (e.g., chronic cor pulmonale), cardiovascular diseases (e.g., heart failure), Liver condition (e.g., cirrhosis, liver cancer)
Secondary blood stasis caused by qi deficiency	Fatigue, lethargy, reluctance to speak, emaciation (Figs. 6-1 and 6-2, 6-4, 6-20 to 6-24)	Malignant conditions (e.g., cancer) chronic condition (e.g., cirrhosis, cachexia)
Tongue and pulse	Dark red or purple in color, with ecchymosis or spots on the tongue body; choppy pulse (Figs. 8-7 to 8-10)	

Acupuncture point selection principles:

Remove the obstruction in the channels and collaterals, regulate the qi activity, and promote the circulation of blood

Point selection:

SP-10, BL-17, SP-6, CV-17, ST-21, CV-6

Manipulation method:

Reducing. For patterns that feature qi deficiency, that is, secondary blood stasis caused by qi deficiency, the even needle movement should be used.

Selection of points for complications:

- Qi deficiency: CV-6 with moxibustion, GV-20, LU-9
- Qi stagnation in the Liver and Gallbladder: GB-34, BL-18, PC-6, LR-3
- Chest pain: PC-6, PC-7, LU-7, BL-13, BL-14
- Abdominal distention and pain: LI-4, TB-6, ST-36
- Painful menstruation: CV-4, CV-5, ST-36, SP-6
- Pain caused by physical injury: LI-4, LU-3, GV-26 (when necessary), and local or *ashi* points

Table 6-2: *Acupuncture treatment*

Points	Point Explanation	Point Combinations
SP-10	As a "sea of blood" point, this is very efficient for regulating the blood and removing blood stasis.	
BL-17	The influential point of the blood, this is used to treat different types of blood disorders. Located at the juncture of the upper and middle burners, it can regulate the qi in both burners.	The combination of these three points is frequently used for regulating the blood and harmonizing the blood and qi.
SP-6	Used to nourish the yin and blood, as it is the meeting point of the three foot yin channels and thus improves (or regulates) the circulation of blood and helps prevent blood stasis.	

—continued next page

Points	Point Explanation	Point Combinations
CV-17	An influential point of the qi, it is efficient in regulating the directional flow of the qi both locally and generally throughout the body and is commonly used for stagnation of qi in the chest.	The combination of these three points promotes the function of the Triple Burner.
ST-21	Regulates the qi activities of the Stomach and Spleen and removes obstruction from the middle burner.	
CV-6	Tonifies and regulates the qi of the body.	

Treatment principle:

Regulate the blood and remove blood stasis

Table 6-3: *Treatment with herbal formulas*

HERB AND DOSAGE	FLAVORS AND NATURE	ASSOCIATED CHANNELS	FORMULA ANALYSIS
■ Four-Substance Decoction with Safflower and Peach Pit *(táo hóng sì wù tāng)*			
FOR REMOVING BLOOD STASIS IN THE BODY			
Persicae Semen *(táo rén)*, 6g	Bitter and neutral	Heart and Liver	Both substances are excellent for removing obstruction from the channels and collaterals.
Carthami Flos *(hóng huā)*, 4g	Acrid and warm	Heart and Liver	
Rehmanniae Radix preparata *(shú dì huáng)*, 15g	Sweet and slightly warm	Heart, Liver, and Kidney	Nourishes the blood and yin
Angelicae sinensis Radix *(dāng guī)*, 12g	Sweet, acrid, and warm	Liver and Heart	Nourishes the blood and dispels blood stasis; also good for alleviating pain and regulating the period
Chuanxiong Rhizoma *(chuān xiōng)*, 8g	Acrid and warm	Liver and Gallbladder	Removes blood stasis and improves the circulation of qi
Paeoniae Radix alba *(bái sháo)*, 10g	Sour and cold	Liver and Spleen	Nourishes the blood and yin

Drive out Blood Stasis in the Mansion of Blood Decoction *(xuè fŭ zhú yū tāng)*

FOR TREATING HEADACHE OR CHEST PAIN CAUSED BY BLOOD STASIS

HERB AND DOSAGE	FLAVORS AND NATURE	ASSOCIATED CHANNELS	FORMULA ANALYSIS
Persicae Semen *(táo rén)*, 12g	Bitter and neutral	Heart and Liver	*Táo hóng sì wù tāng* is used as the base formula to remove blood stasis from the channels and alleviate pain.
Carthami Flos *(hóng huā)*, 9g	Acrid and warm	Heart and Liver	
Rehmanniae Radix *(shēng dì huáng)*, 9g	Sweet and slightly warm	Heart, Liver, and Kidney	
Angelicae sinensis Radix *(dāng guī)*, 9g	Sweet, acrid, and warm	Liver and Heart	
Chuanxiong Rhizoma *(chuān xiōng)*, 5g	Acrid and warm	Liver and Gallbladder	
Paeoniae Radix rubra *(chì sháo)*, 6g	Sour and cold	Liver and Spleen	
Achyranthis bidentatae Radix *(niú xī)*, 9g	Bitter, sour, and neutral	Liver and Kidney	Removes obstruction from the channels
Platycodi Radix *(jié gĕng)*, 5g	Bitter, acrid, and slightly warm	Lung	These herbs promote the qi activity and help to remove blood stasis.
Bupleuri Radix *(chái hú)*, 3g	Bitter, acrid, and slightly cold	Liver and Gallbladder	
Aurantii Fructus *(zhĭ ké)*, 6g	Bitter, acrid, and slightly cold	Spleen and Stomach	
Glycyrrhizae Radix *(gān căo)*, 3g	Sweet and neutral	Heart, Lung, Spleen, and Stomach	Regulates and harmonizes the other herbs

—continued next page

■ Cinnamon Twig and Poria Pill *(guì zhī fú líng wán)*

FOR BLOOD STASIS IN THE UTERUS, PENETRATING AND CONCEPTION VESSELS

<table>
<tr><th>HERB AND DOSAGE</th><th>FLAVORS AND NATURE</th><th>ASSOCIATED CHANNELS</th><th>FORMULA ANALYSIS</th></tr>
<tr><td>Cinnamomi Ramulus (guì zhī)</td><td>Acrid and warm</td><td>Heart, Lung, and Bladder</td><td>Warms the channels to remove blood stasis and regulates menstrual periods</td></tr>
<tr><td>Poria (fú líng), 9g</td><td>Sweet, bland, and neutral</td><td>Heart, Spleen, and Kidney</td><td>Tonifies the qi to help the flow of blood</td></tr>
<tr><td>Moutan Cortex (mǔ dān pí), 9g</td><td>Bitter, acrid, and cold</td><td>Heart, Liver, and Kidney</td><td rowspan="3">Regulates the circulation of blood and removes blood stasis</td></tr>
<tr><td>Persicae Semen (táo rén), 9g</td><td>Bitter and neutral</td><td>Heart and Liver</td></tr>
<tr><td>Paeoniae Radix (sháo yào), 9g</td><td>Bitter and slightly cold</td><td>Liver</td></tr>
</table>

CHAPTER 7

Patterns of Bleeding

Hemorrhage Caused by Hot Blood Patterns

Clinical manifestations

Medical bleeding (not associated with trauma). The bleeding can be caused by various medical conditions and can occur internally or externally. This would include hemoptysis, hematemesis, epistaxis, some acute brain hemorrhaging or retinal hemorrhaging, subcutaneous bleeding (such as ecchymoses or bruising), vaginal bleeding, and hematuria or hematochezia such as lower gastrointestinal bleeding (but not melena).

Key points: See Figs. 7-1 through 7-4 (pp. 118-119).

Pathological process

Bleeding with deep or bright red blood is a characteristic of hemorrhaging caused by a hot blood pattern. As a yang pathogenic factor, the heat accelerates the flow of blood, damages the channels and collaterals, forces blood out of the vessels (channels and collaterals), and finally causes bleeding. In Chinese medicine, this pathological process is called the chaotic movement of hot blood (*xuè rè wàng xíng* 血热妄行).

Blood leaking from damaged channels or collaterals and gathering under the skin (in subcutaneous bleeding) results in bruises. Dense, deep red bruises are a result of blood accumulating in the skin, caused by heat accelerating the circulation of the blood.

Blood vessels can also be damaged by pathogenic heat and internal bleeding, such as in subconjunctival hemorrhage or hematochezia with abdominal pain. Depending on which vessels have been damaged, other types of internal bleeding can also be found clinically.

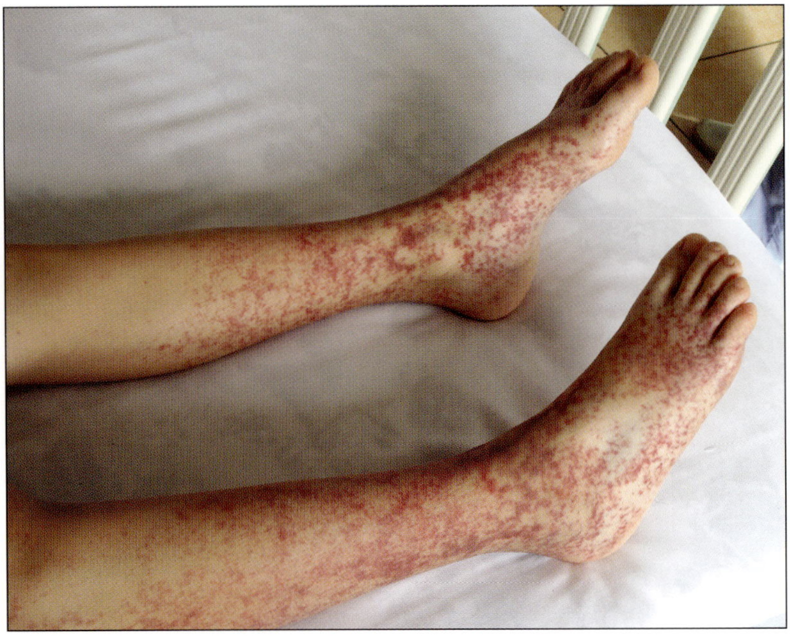

Fig. 7-1: *Henoch-Schōnlein purpura (HSP) or allergic purpura*

Red or purple bruises have developed on the lower legs and feet. The patient complains of abdominal pain accompanied by blood in the stools.

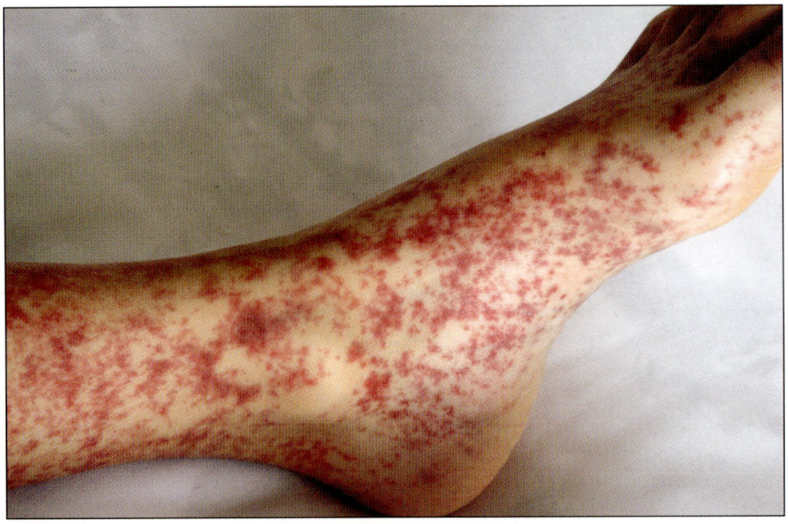

Fig. 7-2: *Same case*

A closer view of the bruises. These are dense, deep red bruises, which do not disappear when pressure is applied to the skin.

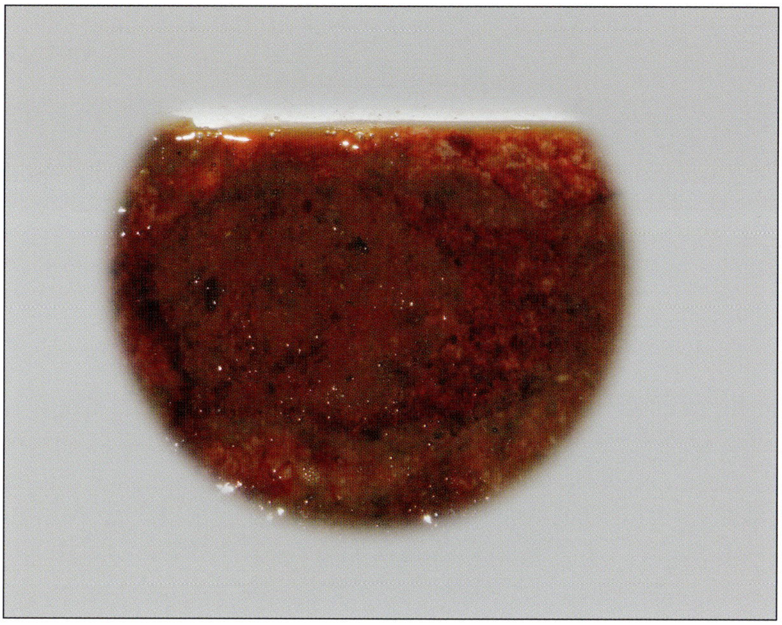

Fig. 7-3: *Ulcerative colitis*

Abdominal pain and diarrhea. The image shows feces mixed with blood and mucus.

(The three images above are the same photos labeled Figs. 4-26 to 4-28 in Ch. 4 on hot blood patterns.)

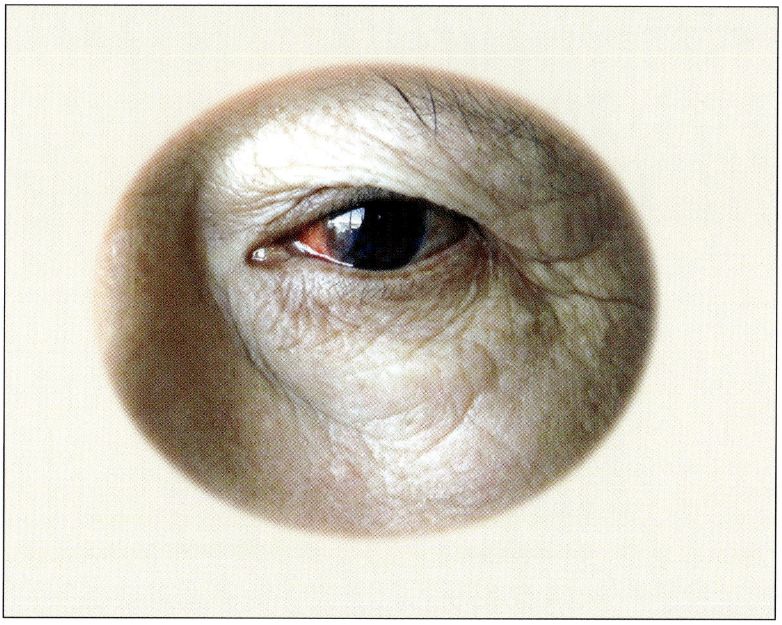

Fig. 7-4: *Subconjunctival hemorrhage associated with high blood pressure*

A bright red patch (or bruise) underneath the conjunctiva in the sclera is observable.

Diagnosis

Hot blood pattern with the chaotic movement of hot blood

The cluster of red or purple bruises indicates a hot blood pattern. The failure of the color to disappear under pressure indicates that the channels have been damaged by heat. Feces mixed with blood indicates that the vessels in the Large Intestine have been damaged.

Differential diagnosis

Hemorrhaging caused by hot blood patterns is very commonly encountered in the clinic. The reason for the hemorrhages seen here is pathogenic heat or fire, which is either heat from excess or deficiency. The excess heat can be due to either an attack by pathogenic factors (heat) in the environment or to a preponderance of yang, which often develops from retention of heat or fire in the organs, such as heat or fire in the Heart or Stomach. On the other hand, heat from deficiency is caused by a deficiency of yin and thus a relative preponderance of yang, such as yin deficiency of the Heart or Kidney. However, the bleeding that results from heat or fire of both excess and deficiency can be bright red, red, or deep red and thick. The main distinguishing points between the two are that hemorrhaging caused by heat or fire from excess is often acute onset with significant blood loss and is a serious condition. By contrast, the symptoms associated with hemorrhaging from the heat or fire of deficiency are less severe because there is less heat, and the type of bleeding can also be different, such as an ongoing low-volume oozing.

Hemorrhage Caused by Qi Deficiency Patterns

Clinical manifestations

Hemorrhages such as subcutaneous bleeding (usually with a scarcity of petechiae), gingival hemorrhage, menorrhagia, gastrointestinal hemorrhage, with pale or sallow, weak, and lusterless appearance. Patients complain of shortness of breath, dizziness, fatigue, and tiredness. A massive blood loss with pale and clammy skin indicates a serious condition called devastated yang (*wáng yáng* 亡阳), which means a serious deficiency or loss of qi and yang in the body.

Key points: See Fig. 7-5 (p. 121).

Pathological process

Subcutaneous bleeding indicates that the blood has leaked from the vessels into the surrounding tissue.

In Chinese medicine the Spleen governs the blood, that is, it controls the blood circulating within the vessels, preventing it from leaking. When the Spleen qi or Spleen yang is deficient, its ability to control the blood is affected such that the blood even-

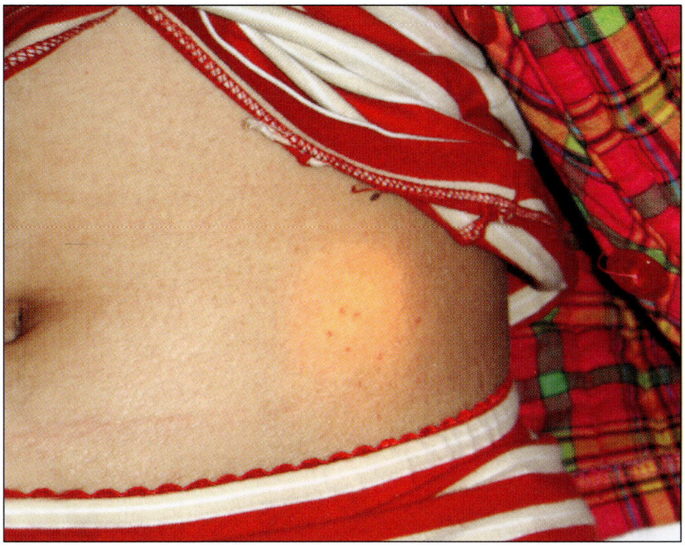

Fig. 7-5: *Idiopathic thrombocytopenic purpura (ITP)*

A small group of pinpoint light red spots (petechiae) have appeared in the illuminated area of skin on the abdomen. The color of the petechiae does not disappear after pressure is applied to the area and the skin is pale and lusterless. (This is the same photo shown in Ch. 2 [Fig. 2-19] on patterns of qi and Spleen deficiency.)

tually leaks out of the vessels under the skin, causing bleeding. This is known as the Spleen being unable to govern the blood (*pí bù tǒng xuè* 脾不统血).

Because the Spleen qi is deficient, its transportive and transformative functions are impaired. Pale and lusterless skin reveals insufficient production of food essence and therefore the malnourishment of the skin. Qi deficiency leads to a lack of energy in the body and the patient therefore becomes tired and fatigued.

Diagnosis

Qi deficiency and dysfunction of the Spleen in governing the blood

Pale, lusterless skin indicates malnourishment of the skin. Fatigue and tiredness reflect Spleen qi deficiency. Subcutaneous bleeding and recurrent hemorrhaging indicate dysfunction of the Spleen's ability to govern the blood.

Differential diagnosis

In Chinese medicine, subcutaneous bleeding (petechiae) has a special name, *jī nǜ* 肌衄, which means "bleeding in the muscles." Subcutaneous bleeding in this case is due to the Spleen's inability to govern the blood, which is caused by Spleen deficiency. It also appears in patterns of hot blood. The purpura occur due to pathogenic heat entering the blood level and accelerating the circulation of the blood, causing it to flow faster and to break out of the channels and collaterals into the surrounding tissue. In Chinese medicine this is known as the chaotic movement of hot blood.

The differences between the two patterns are as follows. The petechiae or purpura caused by pathogenic heat, a pattern of excess, are purple-red or deep red, and the patient's symptoms are associated with hot blood patterns. On the other hand, the petechiae that are caused by the dysfunction of the Spleen in governing the blood, which belongs to deficient or deficient cold patterns, are usually light red to light purple or blue, and the patient's symptoms are associated with Spleen deficiency. (Subcutaneous bleeding is also associated with patterns of blood stasis, and its diagnosis and differentiation can be found in Ch. 6.)

Hemorrhage Caused by Blood Stasis Patterns

Clinical manifestations

These are recurrent hemorrhages, such as subcutaneous bleeding, menorrhagia, hematuria, hematemesis or melena, or bleeding in patients with advanced cancer.

The color of the blood is dark, dark purple or black, and blood clots can be observed. The blood clots are most commonly encountered during heavy menstrual periods. The menstrual blood can be red or dark and thick, with purple or black clots in it. Patients also complain of prolonged or painful menstrual periods.

The formation of blots or spots in the retina, caused by recurrent retinal hemorrhage, also pertain to blood stasis patterns.

Key points: See Figs. 7-6 and 7-7 (below and p. 123).

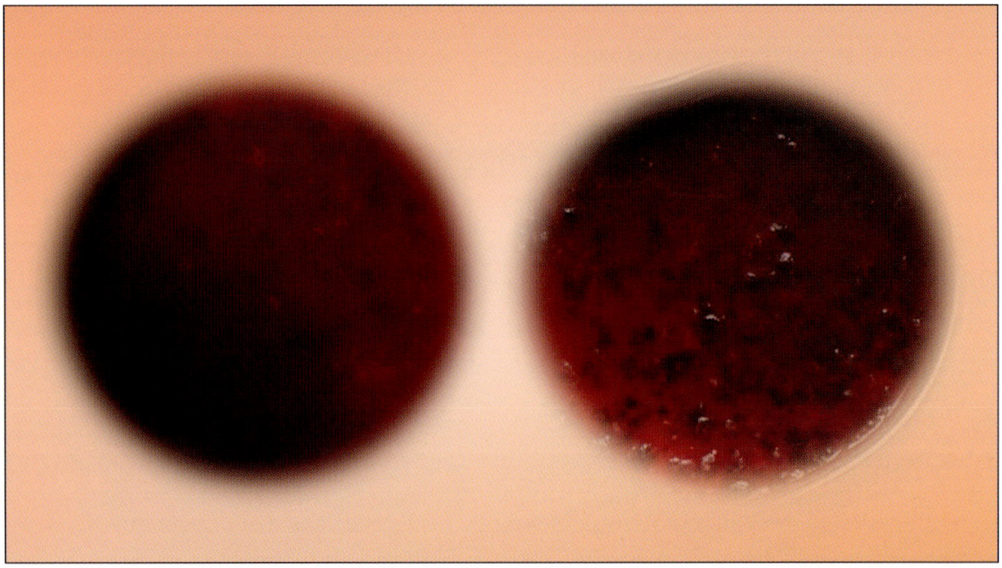

Fig. 7-6: *Irregular period*

A few dark purple or black clots can be seen in the dark red, thick menstrual blood. The patient also complains of sharp lower abdominal pain and dull back pain, beginning several days before and lasting until after the first few days of the onset of the period. (This photo also appears as Fig. 6-19 in Ch. 6 on blood stasis.)

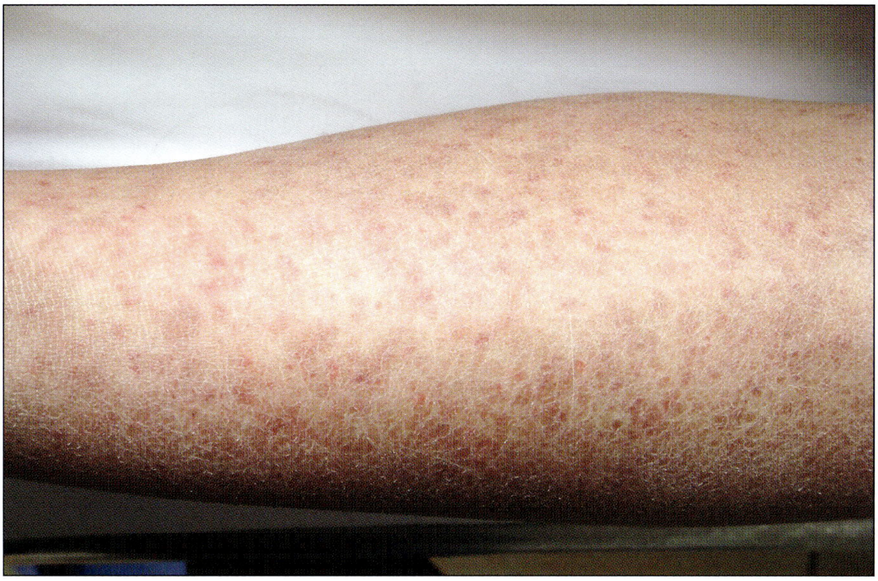

Fig. 7-7: *Henoch-Schönlein purpura (HSP)*

Light purple or blue bruises can be observed on the lower legs, which do not disappear with pressure. There are quite a few bruises but the density is not as great as those in Figs. 7-1 and 7-2.

Pathological process

Dark and thick blood containing blood clots indicates a hemorrhage associated with patterns of blood stasis. Blood clots in the menstrual blood indicate blood stasis in the Penetrating and Conception vessels and in the uterus.

As the flow of blood slows down and accumulates, the color of the blood becomes dark red and the texture turns thick and sticky. This change in the consistency of menstrual blood causes the clots, which are purple or black.

A regular period disturbed by blood stasis in the Penetrating and Conception vessels results in prolonged menstrual periods. In addition, changes in menstrual blood loss can be observed in patients with blood stasis; the menstrual flow varies from scanty to profuse.

When normal circulation of qi and blood is restricted or blocked, physical pain will result. In this case, the blockage has occurred in the uterus, causing the patient to experience painful menstrual periods (dysmenorrhea).

Bleeding can occur in different parts of the body with similar manifestations as those described above and sharing the same pathological process.

According to conventional medicine, there are no great differences between the patients seen in Figs. 7-1 and 7-7 as they both suffer from Henoch-Schönlein purpura (HSP). But in Chinese medicine, different colored bruises and other manifestations imply different causes (or patterns), which require different treatments.

Diagnosis

Blood stasis in the channels and collaterals or uterus

Prolonged and/or painful menstrual periods indicate a blockage of qi and blood in the Penetrating and Conception vessels and/or the uterus. The thick menstrual blood indicates poor blood circulation. The light purple or blue bruises or the dark red clots in the menstrual blood indicate a pattern of blood stasis.

Differential diagnosis

Clots are important diagnostic indicators of blood stasis in cases of hemorrhage, including abnormal menstrual bleeding, obstetrical hemorrhage such as postpartum hemorrhage, gastrointestinal bleeding, or hematuria.

Menstrual disorders caused by blood stasis can result in different symptoms such as scanty menstrual bleeding, a lengthened cycle, an irregular menstrual cycle, and/or dysmenorrhea. Although they have different symptoms, the menstrual blood in these patients shares the same characteristics:

- dark red, dark brown, or black-red menstrual discharge
- sticky or thick discharge
- blood clots.

The symptoms are similar for both patterns of blood stasis in the uterus and pathogenic cold constricting the uterus. (To distinguish between these two patterns, see Ch. 5 on cold blood patterns.)

Summary

For acupuncture and herbal treatment of bleeding patterns, please refer to the relevant chapters.

Table 7-1: *Key diagnostic points for patterns of bleeding*

HEMORRHAGE CAUSED BY PATTERNS OF:

	Hot Blood	Qi Deficiency	Blood Stasis
Images:	Figs. 7-1 to 7-4	Fig. 7-5	Figs. 7-6 and 7-7
Cause of symptoms:	Chaotic movement of hot blood	Inability of the Spleen to govern the blood	Blood stasis in the channels and collaterals
Blood characteristics:	Deep or bright red and thick blood, cluster of purple-red or deep red or purpuric bruises in the skin	Light red to pink and thin or watery blood, pinpoint light red or light blue spots (petechiae) in the skin	Dark red, dark brown or black-red blood, especially in menstrual discharge that is often sticky or thick; dark red, dark purple or black blood clots can be observed; light purpuric or blue bruises in the skin
Symptoms:	Fever, anxiety, restlessness, insomnia; red complexion and skin, thirst, yellow urine, and dry stools	Pale or sallow, weak, and lusterless appearance, shortness of breath, dizziness, fatigue and tiredness, emaciation, poor appetite, and abdominal discomfort	Bluish discoloration (cyanosis) of skin, lips, and fingernails; rough and scaly skin; fixed and sharp pain; firm and hard mass in abdomen
Examples of diseases:	Many different types of internal or external bleeding such as hemoptysis, hematemesis, epistaxis, subcutaneous bleeding, vaginal bleeding, and hematuria or hematochezia such as lower GI bleeding; some brain hemorrhaging or retinal hemorrhaging such as hypertension or diabetes retinopathy	Subcutaneous bleeding (usually with a scarcity of petechiae), gingival hemorrhage, menorrhagia, gastrointestinal hemorrhage, recurrent hemorrhaging	Recurrent hemorrhages such as retinal hemorrhage, subcutaneous bleeding, menorrhagia, hematuria, hematemesis or melena
Tongue and pulse:	Scarlet tongue, rapid pulse	Pale and flabby tongue with teeth marks around the border; forceless pulse	Dark red or purple in color, with spots on the tongue body; choppy pulse

CHAPTER 8

Tongue Diagnosis for Patients with Qi and/or Blood Disorders

Since this book is not specifically devoted to tongue diagnosis, only a few examples of typical tongue changes related to the conditions described in this book are illustrated. For more information about tongue diagnosis methodology and the changes that occur on the tongue, readers should consult illustrated atlases that are dedicated to tongue diagnosis.

The main changes on the tongue (especially the color) due to qi or blood disorders appear on the tongue body. A change in the coating is primarily caused by an invasion of any one or more of the six external pathogenic factors, or by internal pathogenic factors such as phlegm, dampness, or retention of food. In this book, the focus is on qi and blood disorders and therefore these illustrations of tongue changes mainly depict the tongue body; the coating is almost normal or changes very little. The tongue images are grouped together so that they can be easily compared and understood by the reader.

Pale Tongue

Clinical manifestations

The color of the tongue body is paler than that of a normal tongue. The shape of the tongue can be thin and slender, and the tongue coating normal or abnormal, depending on the cause and site of the disease as well as the pathological processes.

Key points: See Figs. 8-1 and 8-2 (p. 128).

Pathological process

The color of the tongue body is directly related to the color of the blood in the vessels. Blood deficiency means an inadequate supply of blood in the channels. Without sufficient circulation of blood, the tongue color becomes paler than normal.

Diagnosis

Patterns of blood deficiency, or of dual qi and blood deficiency

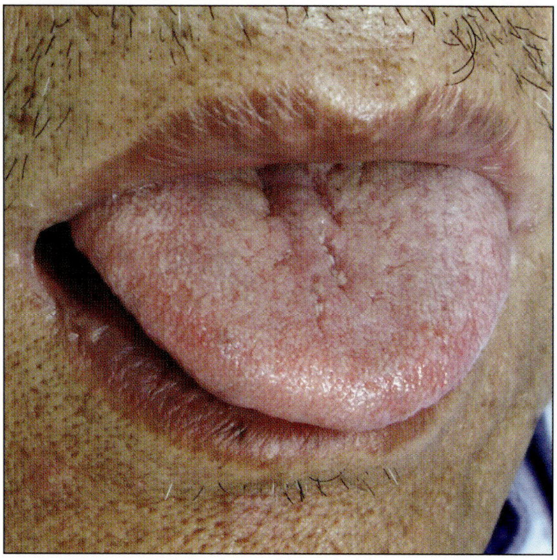

Fig. 8-1: *Anemia due to chronic renal failure*
Pale tongue with a thin and white coating

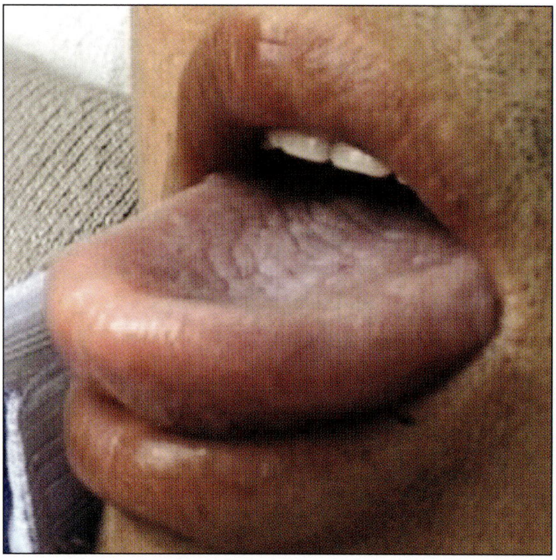

Fig. 8-2: *A patient with iron-deficiency anemia*
Pale and lusterless tongue. The shape of the tongue body is normal and the coating is thin and white.

Pale and Swollen Tongue

Clinical manifestations

Pale, swollen, flabby tongue body with or without teeth marks around the border. The tongue coating is usually white in color, thick and moist, even watery. A greasy and thick coating may also be observed.

Key points: See Figs. 8-3 and 8-4 below.

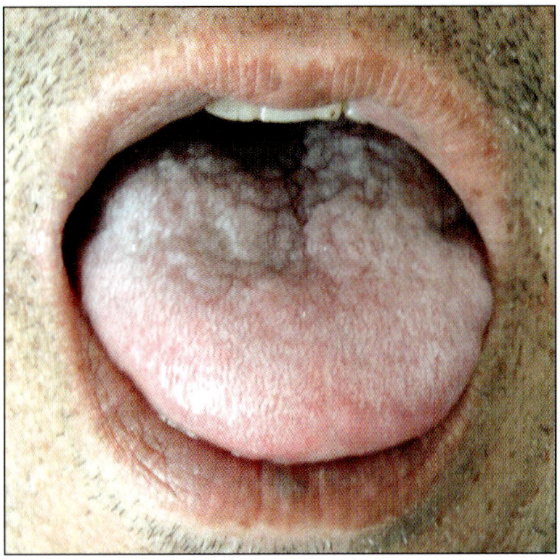

Fig. 8-3: *Chronic cor pulmonale*

Pale, dull, lusterless, and swollen tongue body with white tongue coating. The coating at the middle and root of the tongue is slightly thicker.

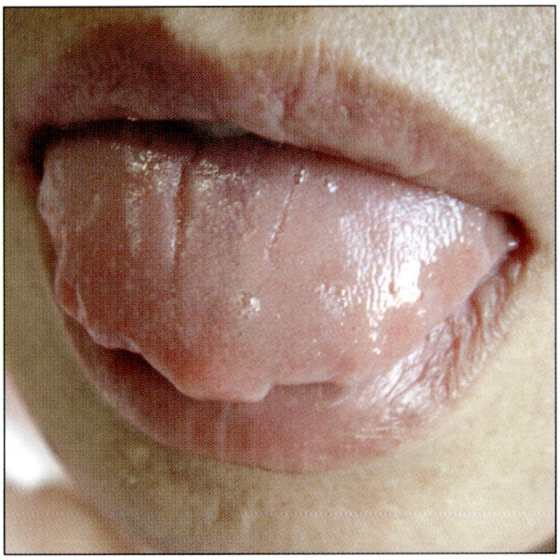

Fig. 8-4: *Kidney failure with uremia*

Pale, soft, and flabby tongue body with obvious teeth marks. The tongue coating is white, watery, and very thin, which indicates a condition of qi and yang deficiency.

Pathological process

There are two causes for this color of the tongue: first, a deficiency of qi leading to a lack of energy to circulate the blood such that the tongue body has insufficient blood circulating within it; and second, Spleen qi deficiency resulting in a dysfunction in the transporting and transforming of food essence such that the blood has insufficient nutrition. Deficiency of Spleen yang can also cause retention of fluids or dampness in the body; as a result, the tongue body may be swollen and flabby with teeth marks around the border and the tongue coating may be more moist than usual.

Diagnosis

This type of tongue indicates qi deficiency, especially a pattern of Spleen qi or Spleen yang deficiency.

Scarlet Tongue

Clinical manifestations

Deep red, purplish, or scarlet coloration with a dry and rough texture. The tongue body may become hard and firm, or very thin and slender. The tongue coating can be thin or thick but is very often dry. In serious cases, a cracked tongue coating can be observed.

Key points: See Figs. 8-5 and 8-6 (below and p. 131).

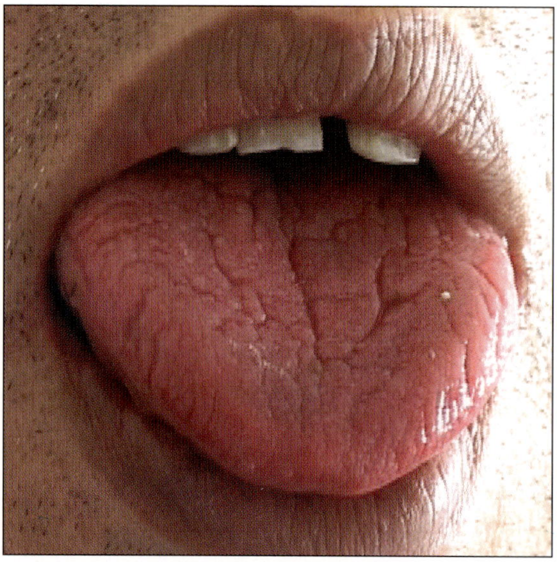

Fig. 8-5: *Acute pneumonia with high temperature*

Red color with an absence of tongue coating. Some cracks can be observed on the tongue body.

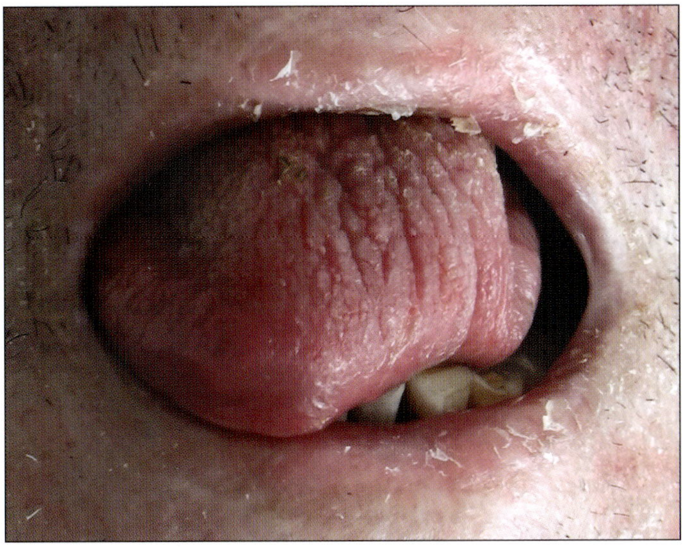

Fig. 8-6: *Serious infection following burn trauma*

Deep red color, very dry, rough, and hard tongue body, with deep cracks. The tongue coating is also very dry.

Pathological process

A scarlet tongue has a deeper hue than that of a red tongue. The deep red or scarlet coloration indicates that heat has reached the nutritive level or blood level and has exacerbated the circulation, causing an accumulation of blood in the channels and collaterals as well as in the tongue body. In addition, pathogenic heat has consumed the body fluids and therefore the tongue body has become dry. On a deeper level, the yin is also consumed and thus there is not enough essence to nourish the tongue body; it therefore appears rough, hard, and even cracked.

Diagnosis

Hot blood patterns

Dark Purple Tongue

Clinical manifestations

Dark purple or bluish tongue coloration. Purple or bluish spots (ecchymosis) may be observed on the surface or border of the tongue. The coating can be any type, but a white and watery coating is most likely to be seen in patients with patterns of cold blood.

Key points: See Figs. 8-7 through 8-10 (pp. 132-133).

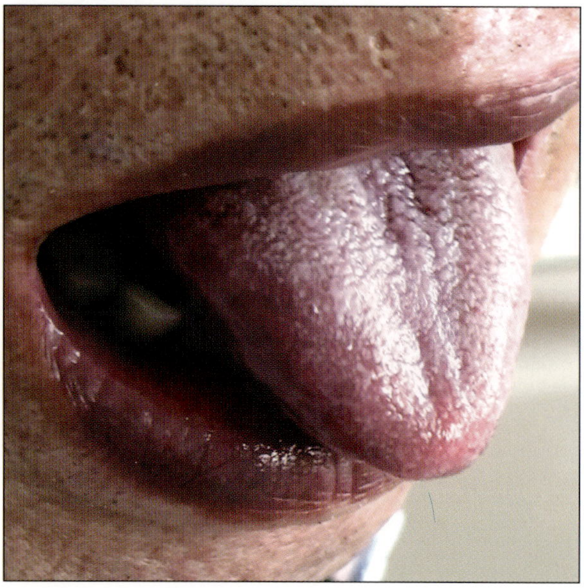

Fig. 8-7: *A patient with chronic cor pulmonale*
Dark purple, lusterless tongue with a thin and white coating

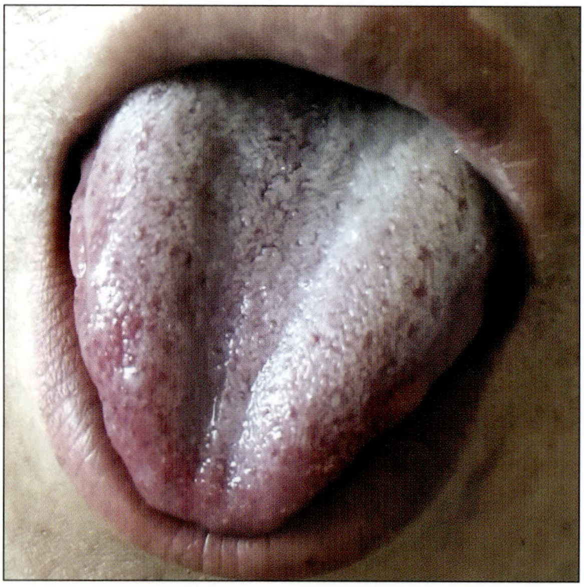

Fig. 8-8: *Heart failure*

Dark purple, lusterless tongue with a thick, white, and moist coating indicating that there is a pathological process related to pathogenic cold congealing the blood in the channels and blood stasis obstructing the vessels; in other words, a cold blood pattern

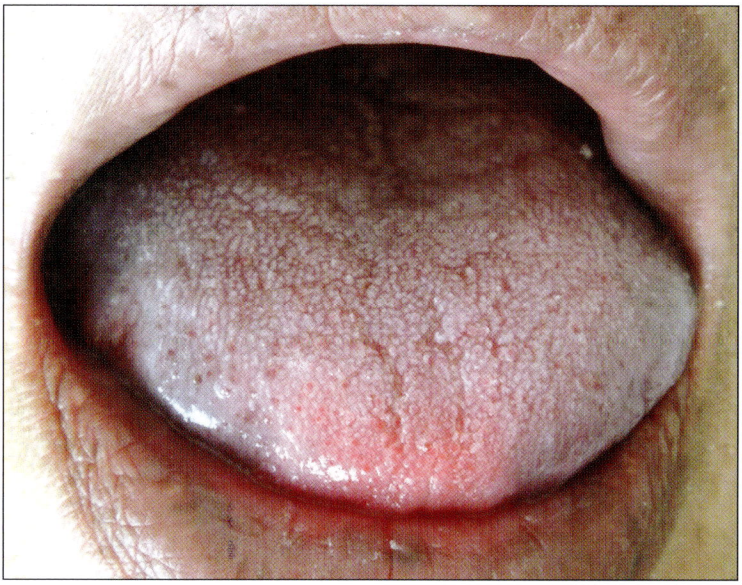

Fig. 8-9: *Diabetes*

There are large bluish bruises on both borders of the tongue body.

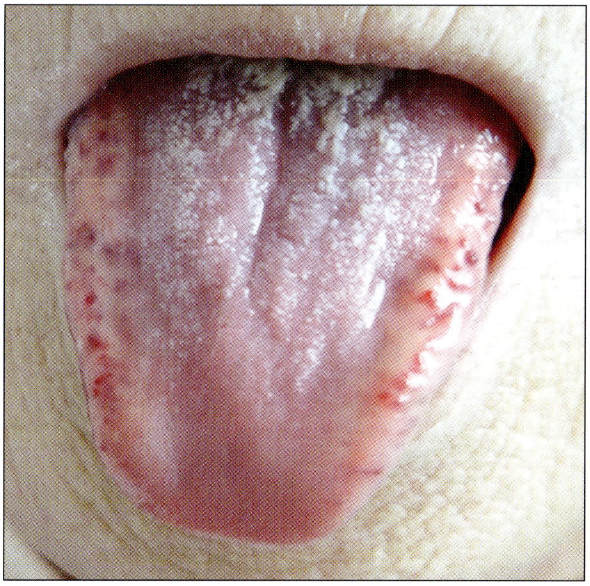

Fig. 8-10: *Ischemic stroke*

This is a pale tongue with small purple spots on the borders of the body and a white, thick, and greasy coating at the root of the tongue.

Pathological process

Blood stasis is a dysfunction of blood circulation in the channels and collaterals. Spots (ecchymosis) or a dark red color appear on the tongue body indicating that the flow of blood is slowing down in the tongue as well as in the body; this is blood stasis. The lack of luster on the tongue indicates a failure of yang qi to reach the surface of the body due to an obstruction caused by blood stasis.

Diagnosis

This tongue can be viewed as a manifestation of two types of patterns: blood stasis and cold blood.

Cold blood patterns are caused by pathogenic cold, which involves a retention of dampness or pathogenic body fluids in the body. Thus we can also see a moist tongue coating as well as a dark purple tongue body.

Blood stasis patterns can have various causes such as qi stagnation or qi deficiency. In the latter case, besides symptoms of blood stasis, there is also qi deficiency and thus the tongue is flabby and may have teeth marks around the border (as shown in Fig. 8-4), with a dark, purple, or blue coloration.

Normal Tongue

Clinical manifestations

Light red, lustrous tongue body with normal shape and suppleness in movement and a thin, white, and slightly moist coating. According to Chinese medical theory, a normal tongue is thought to have "normal spirit."

Key points: See Fig. 8-11 below.

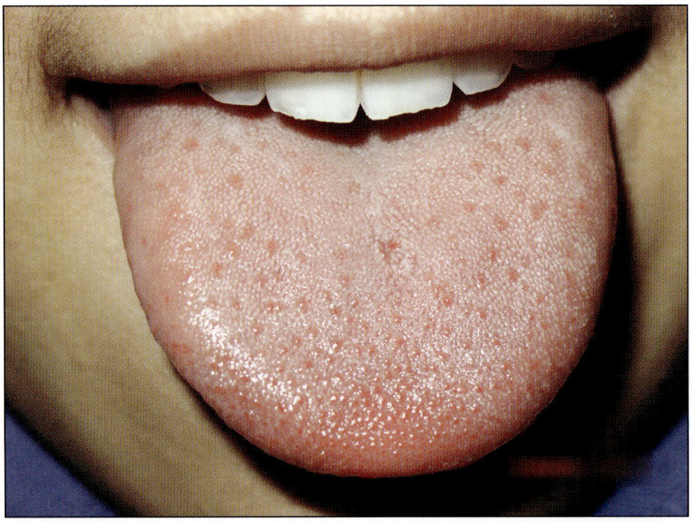

Fig. 8-11: *A normal tongue body and tongue coating*

Diagnosis

A healthy person with sufficient qi and blood supply, or a slightly sick person, which means that the antipathogenic factors have not yet been damaged, such as seen in an exterior pattern.

Key Points of Comparison for the Tongue

The practitioner should pay special attention to the following points:

- Color: Different colors indicate different patterns.
- Luster: The luster of a normal tongue can decrease or disappear completely, depending on the severity of damage to the antipathogenic factors.
- Moisture on the tongue signifies that the body fluids are not injured. With cold patterns (such as Spleen yang deficiency or cold blood), the tongue and tongue coating can be more moist or even watery because of retention of water in the body, but with heat patterns, the heat consumes the body fluids and thereby causes the tongue to become dry.
- Texture: A soft and smooth appearance of the tongue body requires a sufficient supply of nutrition and fluids. In cases involving cold patterns, retention of pathogenic water or dampness can cause the tongue to become swollen or flabby. With heat patterns, the tongue body can look dull, rough, and hard following dehydration caused by pathogenic heat consuming the blood and body fluids.

APPENDIX

Additional Information on Qi and Blood

Qi and Blood in the Human Body

In Chinese medical theory, qi and blood are the fundamental elements of the human body. The physiological functions of the qi and blood are to provide nutrition and energy in order to support life. Specifically, blood pertains to the yin aspect and all the nourishment needed by the organs is provided by the blood. Qi, which includes qi and yang, pertains to the yang aspect and the energy within the body comes from qi. In addition to their own functions, the qi and blood also depend on each other and transform into each other.

Each of the organs has a yin and a yang aspect. The yang aspect controls the functional activity and the yin aspect governs the substance of the organ itself. Both of these yin and yang aspects are supported by qi (yang) and blood (yin). In other words, sufficient qi and blood are essential to maintain the normal functions of the organs.

Disorders of Qi and/or Blood

The disorders of qi or blood can be caused by a variety of factors and present with different symptoms. Deficiency of qi or blood often produces an appearance of malnutrition or weakness such as pale skin or bodily emaciation. Poor circulation of qi or blood will most likely manifest as local symptoms such as a red or bluish coloration on the skin or as an altered sensation. Dysfunction of qi or blood may cause some serious symptoms such as a prolapse of the organs or edema.

As the qi and blood circulate internally throughout the body, as well as on the body surface, through the channels and collaterals, a disorder of qi or blood can either be manifested externally or internally. When the organs have been affected, symptoms associated with the organs will appear. Examples include Spleen qi deficiency or Heart blood deficiency.

Because there is a symbiotic relationship between the qi and blood, they are interdependent. As a result, a disorder in one can easily upset the other; disorders of both are thus commonly seen in the clinic. For example, a problem such as blood stasis (an obstruction in the channels and collaterals) reduces the flow of the qi and causes qi stagnation.

Diagnosis of Qi and Blood Disorders

When approaching an individual with a disorder of qi or blood, the special differentiation of qi and blood method is used. This diagnosis is based on qi and blood theory. The patient's signs and symptoms are collected and used to ascertain the condition and functional circumstances of qi and blood in order to reach a correct conclusion.

Patterns associated with deficiency of the qi or blood are blood deficiency patterns, qi deficiency patterns, patterns of dual qi and blood deficiency, and qi or blood deficiency patterns involving one or more particular organs or channels or collaterals.

Patterns associated with the obstruction of the qi or blood circulation are blood stasis patterns, qi stagnation patterns, and secondary blood stasis patterns caused by qi stagnation or qi deficiency.

Patterns associated with a dysfunction of the qi or blood are hot blood patterns, cold blood patterns, patterns of reversing qi (in which the qi circulates in the wrong direction), and qi-sinking patterns.

Finally, patterns associated with hemorrhaging are those caused by hot blood, blood stasis, and Spleen qi deficiency (in which the Spleen qi loses its ability to control the blood).

The key points in diagnosing these patterns are summarized at the end of each chapter in this book.

Treatment Principles for Qi and/or Blood Disorders

The treatments listed in the summary charts at the end of each chapter include treatment principles, a selection of acupuncture points, and examples of herbal formulas for treating the various patterns.

Generally speaking, to establish an appropriate treatment, we follow these steps:

- *Make a correct diagnosis.* Based on pattern differentiation, it will be clear why the disorder occurs, whether the disease involves the channels, collaterals, or organs, and whether the antipathogenic factors have been injured. Choose a suitable method or methods of treatment such as acupuncture, moxibustion, cupping, herbal medicine, or other Chinese medical treatment.
- *Select acupuncture points.* This includes choosing the appropriate channels, selecting points or point combinations (local or distant points, or points according to specific point theories) as well as manipulation style, such as the depth and needling direction.

Unlike Chinese herbs and other treatment modalities, acupuncture points have bidirectional regulatory functions, that is, one point can produce a completely different or even opposite result depending on the condition of the body, the manipulation method, and its combination with different points.

For example, GV-14 is a point commonly used in the clinic. This point can be used for expelling external pathogenic factors, especially yang pathogenic factors, and removing heat in the treatment of heat patterns. It also tonifies (reinforces) qi or promotes the yang to treat internal cold caused by a deficiency of yang qi, which means an increase of body heat. In cases of the common cold, the patient's rising temperature implies a condition of heat retention. GV-14 is used to clear this heat. LI-4 is a good choice to combine with it and the reducing method is used. For patients with yang deficiency in whom the body has insufficient energy and heat, GV-14 can also be used to promote the yang qi, but in this instance, it is combined with GV-20 and the tonification method is used.

In the clinic, arriving at a correct diagnosis and devising a suitable treatment is a complicated and mutable procedure. It is based on the foundation of Chinese medical theory, correct differentiation, and the practitioner's personal clinical experience. The patient's individual characteristics, such as age, constitution, social environment (including the psychological constitution, personality, and relationship between colleagues, friends, and family), as well as the natural environment (season and locale), must be taken into account before a treatment can be started.

This book only lists basic treatments, commonly used acupuncture points, and some combinations of acupuncture points, herbs, and formulas. In addition to the principles outlined in this book, one should bear in mind that individual general conditions as well as the reaction to the treatment are variable, and that flexibility is necessary to accommodate the different cases that one encounters in the clinic. Only complete mastery of the basic principles of differentiation can guarantee success in the clinic.

INDEX

A

C

.... E

F

G

H

O

P

Q

R

S

T

Y